Surgery and Y

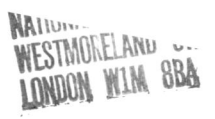

Donald Ross
DSc, FRCS, FACS
Consultant Surgeon, National Heart and Middlesex Hospitals, Director, Department of Surgery, Institute of Cardiology, London

Barbara Hyams
BSc, MA

BEACONSFIELD PUBLISHERS
Beaconsfield, Bucks, England

First published in 1982

This book is copyright under the Berne Convention. All rights are reserved. Apart from any fair dealing for the purpose of private study, research, criticism or review, as permitted under the Copyright Act 1956, no part of this publication may be reproduced, stored in a retrieval system, or transmitted, in any form or by any means, electronic, electrical, chemical, mechanical, optical, photocopying, recording or otherwise, without the prior permission of the copyright owner. Enquiries should be addressed to the Publishers at 20 Chiltern Hills Road, Beaconsfield, Bucks HP9 1PL, England.

Copyright © Donald N. Ross, Barbara E. Hyams, 1982

British Library Cataloguing in Publication Data

Ross, Donald N.
  Surgery and your heart.
  1. Heart—Diseases
  I.Title   II. Hyams, Barbara E.
  616.1'2   RC681

ISBN 0–906584–07–8

Typeset in 10½ on 12 point Times (C.A.T.),
printed and bound in Great Britain
by Billing and Sons Limited,
London, Oxford, Worcester

Contents

	PREFACE	iv
1	**THE STRUCTURE AND FUNCTION OF THE HEART**	1
	The Heart – Outside and Inside	1
	The Chambers of the Heart	4
	The Circulation of the Blood	7
	The Valves of the Heart	10
	The Arteries of the Heart (Coronary Arteries)	12
2	**DISEASES OF THE HEART**	13
	Congenital Heart Disease	
	Simple Defects	13
	Holes in the septa: atrial septal defect and ventricular septal defect	13
	Narrowings in arteries: pulmonary stenosis and coarctation of the aorta	16
	Abnormal connections: patent ductus arteriosus	19
	Complex Defects	20
	Tetralogy of Fallot	20
	Transposition of the great arteries	24
	Acquired Diseases of the Heart	
	Coronary Heart Disease and Heart Attacks	29
	Angina	30
	Heart attack	32
	Aneurysm	34
	Diseases of the Valves	35
	Causes of valve disease	35
	Stenosis of the valves	39
	Regurgitation of the mitral or aortic valves	41
	Multiple valve disease	41
	Valve replacement	43
3	**SPECIAL INVESTIGATIONS**	46
	The X-ray	46
	The Electrocardiogram	47
	The Echocardiogram	48
	Cardiac Catheterization and Angiocardiography	49
4	**THE OPEN HEART OPERATION AND RECOVERY**	52
	The Open Heart Operation	52
	After the Operation	52
	Post-Operative Programme	54
	The first ten days	54
	The three-month convalescent period	57
	Eating, drinking and smoking	57

Preface

In dealing with a large number of patients facing the prospect of an operation upon their heart, I have often been impressed by their unquestioning faith in their medical advisers. At the same time, I have been concerned by their lack of knowledge of the structure and function of that important organ, and the underlying principles of the proposed surgical correction.

I have consequently tried to lay out, in simple language, a brief description of the mechanics of the normal heart, what is likely to go wrong, how we investigate the problems and then set about correcting them.

This booklet aims to present the picture as simply as possible, avoiding technical terms and jargon. It is hoped that it will help the patient, the family and the medical team to come together on common ground. In this endeavour I have been helped by the enthusiasm and expert artistic work of my collaborator, Barbara Hyams.

I am indebted to Bentley Laboratories for supporting this project.

D.N.R.

Chapter 1

The Structure and Function of the Heart

The Heart – Outside and Inside

The heart lies within the chest cavity, with one lung on each side of it. Blood from all parts of the body flows into the heart through blood vessels

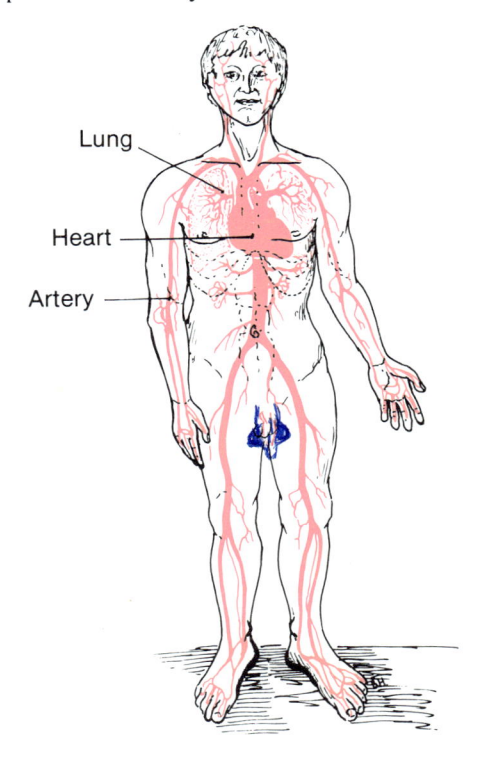

Figure 1 The position of the heart, in the centre of the chest cavity, with the lungs (dotted red lines) on each side of it, and the main arteries of the body. The veins, which are not shown here, run alongside most of the arteries.

Surgery and Your Heart

called veins. As the blood leaves the veins and enters the heart, it is pumped through the lungs and again returns to the heart to be pumped out to the rest of the body through another set of tubes called arteries. This circulation of the blood brings oxygen and nourishment to all parts of the body, and carries waste products away. Figure 1 shows the heart, the lungs (outlined) and the main arteries of the body.

Figure 2 is a drawing which shows the outside of the heart as seen by the surgeon when he looks at the patient's chest from the front. The main body of the heart is the part which acts as a pump. The large tubes are the arteries and veins which carry the blood into and away from the heart.

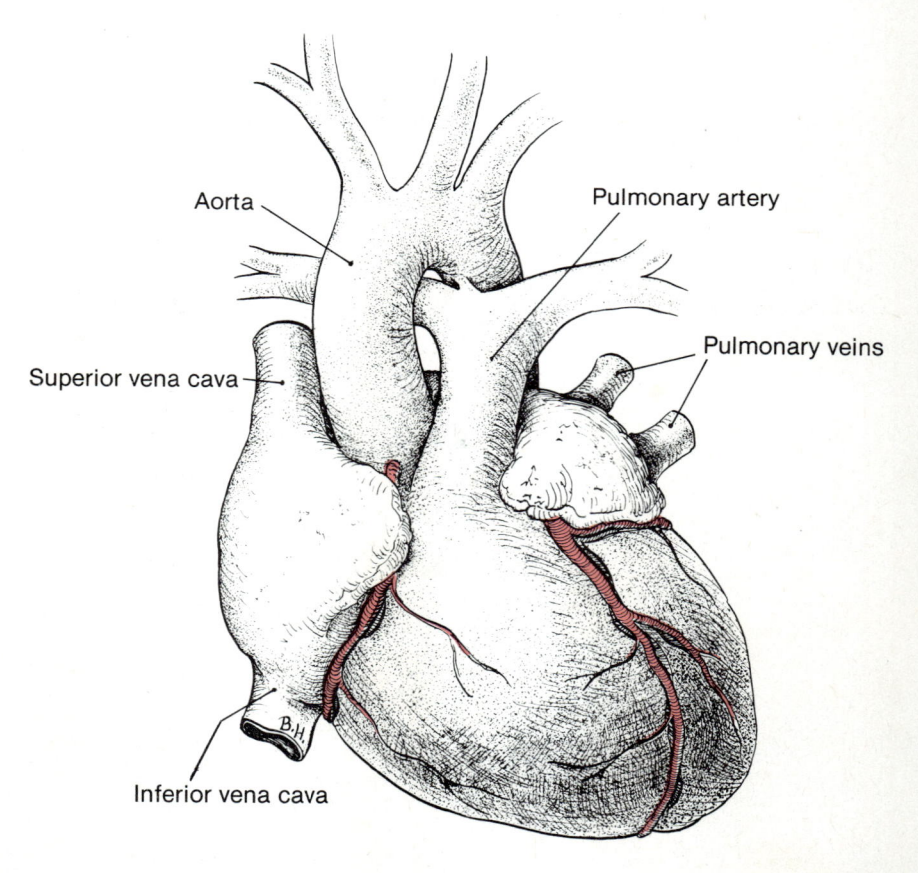

Figure 2   The outside of the heart as seen from the front.

The Structure and Function of the Heart

Figure 3 shows what the heart looks like if it is cut open along its length. You can see that there are four chambers (1, 2, 3 and 4 in the diagram) and two large arteries (A and B). The heart is divided into left and right sides by walls called septa, and on each side there are two chambers and one large artery. Each side has two valves as well, which allow the blood to flow in only one direction.

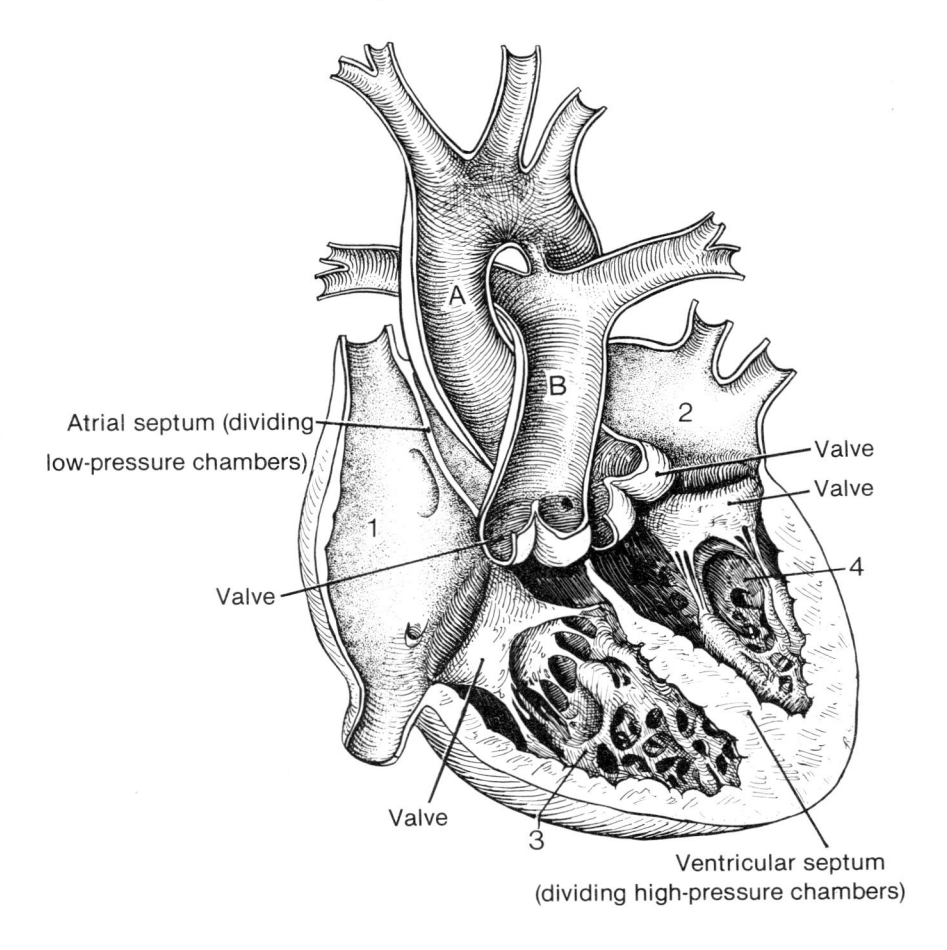

Figure 3 The heart has been cut in half along its length and the top part removed. The four chambers are numbered 1, 2, 3, 4, and the two large arteries that carry blood away from the heart are lettered A, B. There are four valves in the heart.

3

Surgery and Your Heart

Figure 4 is a simplified diagram of Figure 3, again showing the four chambers with the valves leading to the pumping chambers or ventricles, and to the great arteries. This diagram will be used throughout the booklet as a model to show how the heart works, and later, to illustrate the various diseases.

The Chambers of the Heart

The two upper chambers of the heart are called the right and left atria. The atria receive blood coming into the heart and pass this blood to the lower thick-walled chambers, which are called the right and left ventricles. The ventricles are the pumping chambers, and they have thick muscular walls which contract to squeeze the blood out of the heart.

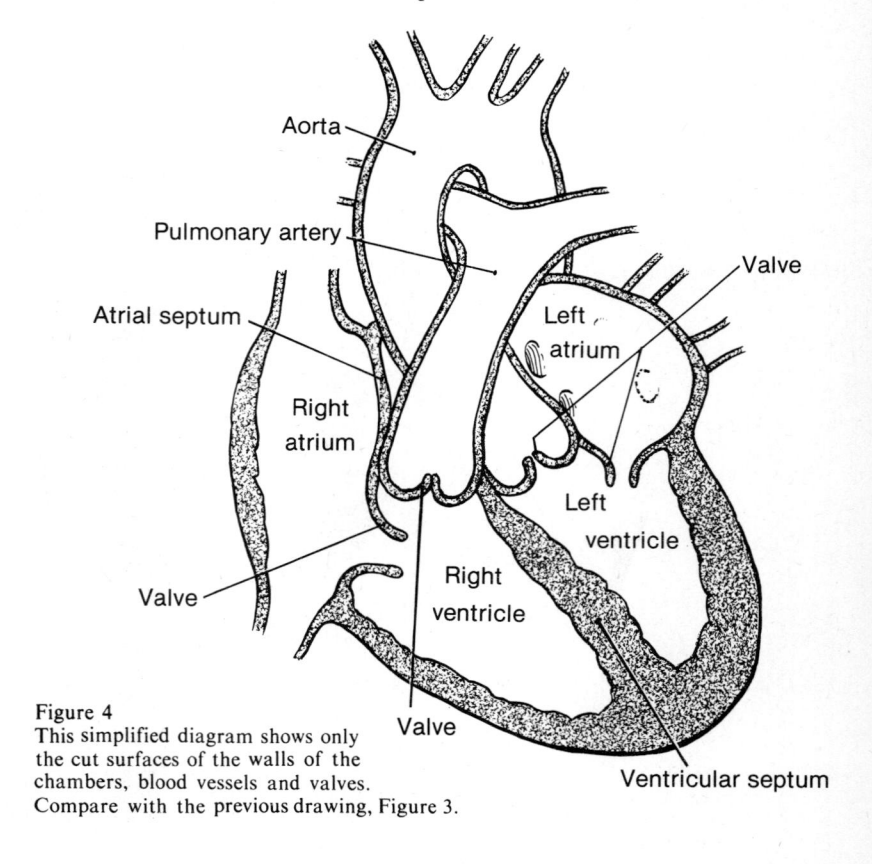

Figure 4
This simplified diagram shows only the cut surfaces of the walls of the chambers, blood vessels and valves. Compare with the previous drawing, Figure 3.

The Structure and Function of the Heart

The heart is divided into right and left sides by the septa (atrial septum and ventricular septum). On each side the blood enters the upper collecting chambers (the atria) through the veins, flows to the lower pumping chambers (the ventricles), and is pumped out through the large arteries connected to the ventricles (aorta and pulmonary artery, Fig. 4).

The right side of the heart receives dark, blue blood which is returning from the body. This blood has delivered its oxygen to the tissues and has collected waste products which must be removed. Because this blood now has very little oxygen in it, it is blue in colour. Blue blood is also called venous blood, because it travels to the heart through the veins.

The venous blood from the head, neck, arms, legs, and organs enters the right atrium (RA) through two large veins (Figure 5). It passes into

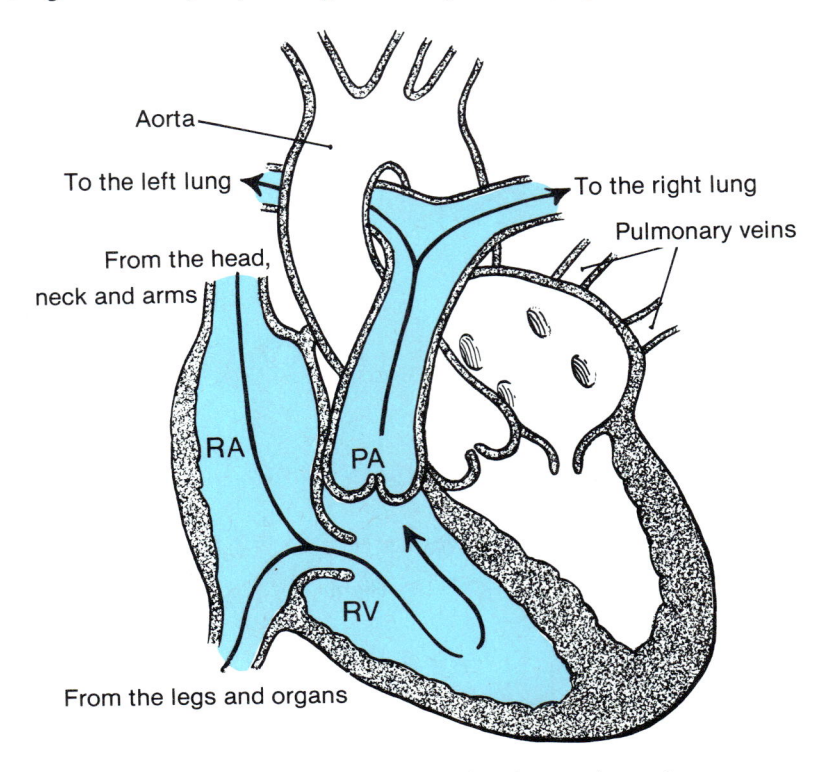

Figure 5 The blue blood from the head, neck, arms, legs and organs enters the right atrium (RA) through two large veins. It flows into the right ventricle (RV), and is pumped out to the lungs through the pulmonary artery (PA).

Surgery and Your Heart

the right ventricle (RV) and, from here, is pumped out of the heart through the pulmonary artery (PA). The pulmonary artery carries the blue blood to the lungs.

In the lungs the blue venous blood gives up its waste products. It also receives a fresh supply of oxygen, which changes its colour from blue to bright red. This 'oxygenated' red blood returns to the left side of the heart through the pulmonary veins, which bring the red blood into the left atrium (LA, Figure 6).

The red blood collected in the left atrium then flows to the left ventricle (LV) and is pumped under considerable pressure through the large artery called the aorta. This pressure drives the blood through the head, neck, arms, legs and various organs of the body, and is responsible for our blood pressure.

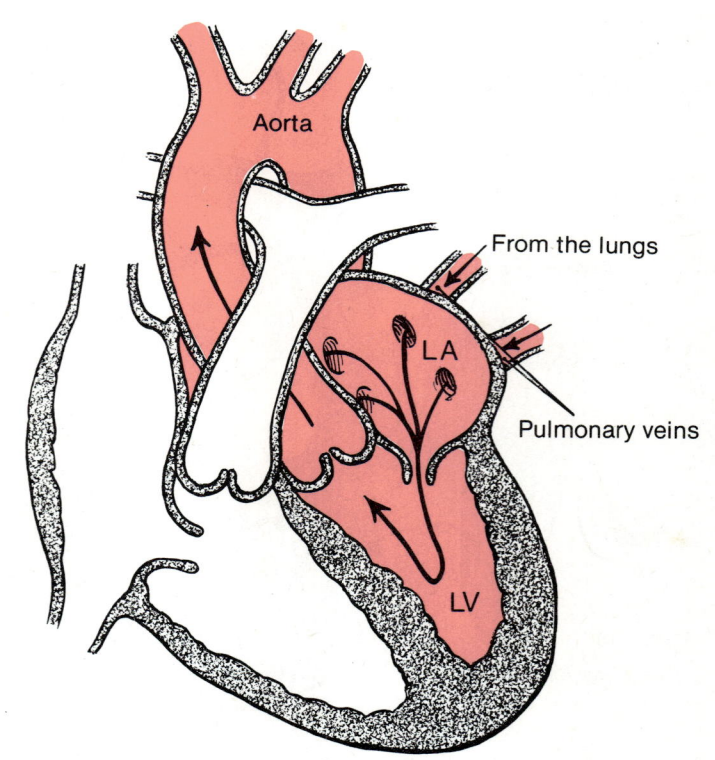

Figure 6 The red blood returns from the lungs by the pulmonary veins, enters the left atrium (LA) and flows into the left ventricle (LV). From here it is pumped out to the body through the aorta.

6

The Structure and Function of the Heart

The Circulation of the Blood

We will now consider one complete cycle of the blood's circulation.

The right ventricle (RV) receives the blue blood from the right atrium (RA) and pumps it into the pulmonary artery (Figure 7). The pulmonary artery branches into two above the heart, so that half of the blood flows to the right lung and half goes to the left lung. Within the lungs, the pulmonary arteries branch again like a tree to form many little arteries. These arteries continue to branch until they form microscopic blood vessels, so small that only one blood cell at a time can enter them. These very tiny blood vessels are called capillaries, and it is in these capillaries that the blood is able to interact with the air in the lungs and exchange waste products from the body for a fresh supply of oxygen. After a short distance the capillaries connect to form tiny veins. These veins in turn join together to form larger veins, and eventually become the pulmonary veins which carry the red oxygen-rich blood to the left atrium of the heart.

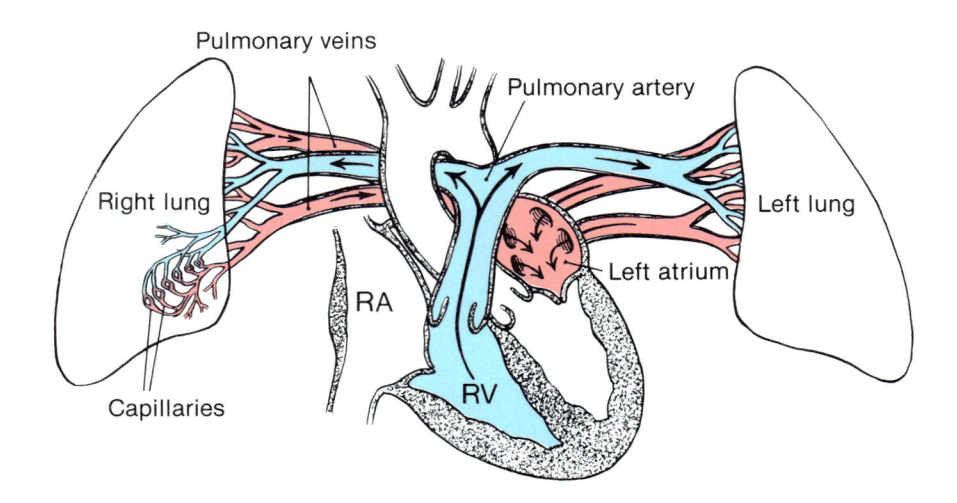

Figure 7 The circulation of the blood in the lungs. Blue blood is pumped through the pulmonary arteries to the lungs, where it absorbs oxygen in the tiny capillaries surrounding the air cells of the lung, and returns to the heart as red blood through the pulmonary veins.

Surgery and Your Heart

The red oxygenated blood flows from the left atrium to the left ventricle, and the left ventricle pumps this red blood out of the heart through the aorta (Figure 8). The aorta branches into smaller arteries, which carry the red blood to all parts of the body. The oxygen in this blood is distributed to all of the body's tissues, and in exchange the blood collects all of the waste products. Just as in the lungs, this exchange occurs in the tiny capillaries which connect all of the small arteries to all the small veins of the body. As the oxygen is gradually used up by the tissue cells, the colour of the blood becomes blue. The blue blood collects in the veins of the body and returns to the right atrium of the heart. This completes one full cycle of the circulation.

The Structure and Function of the Heart

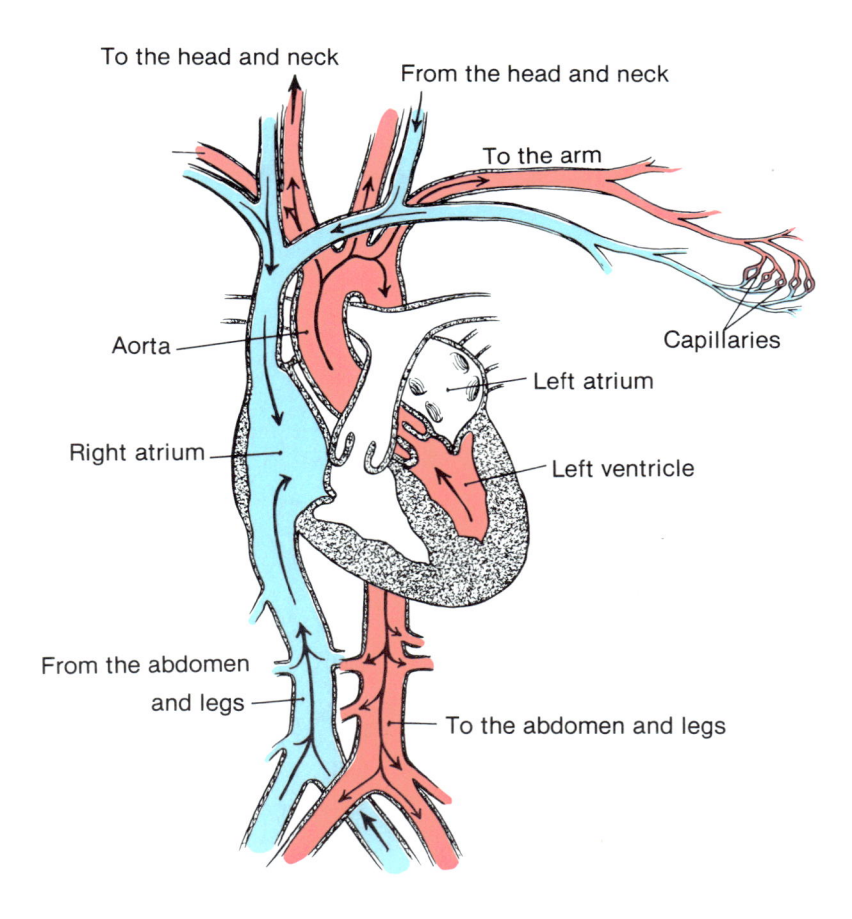

Figure 8 The circulation of the oxygenated blood through the body. The red blood leaves the heart through the aorta and is distributed to all the blood vessels in the head, neck, arms, legs and organs. The blood exchanges oxygen for waste products in the tiny capillaries, and returns to the heart through veins as blue (venous) blood.

Surgery and Your Heart

The Valves of the Heart

In order to ensure that the blood flows in only one direction when the heart contracts, there are four one-way valves which act like doors within the heart (Figure 9). The two valves which control the flow of blood into and out of the left ventricle are the most important valves in the heart. These are called the mitral and aortic valves (Figure 9). The corresponding but less important valves on the right side are called the tricuspid and pulmonary valves.

These valves work in a simple way, rather like doors. When blood moves through them in a forward direction, the flaps of the valves open.

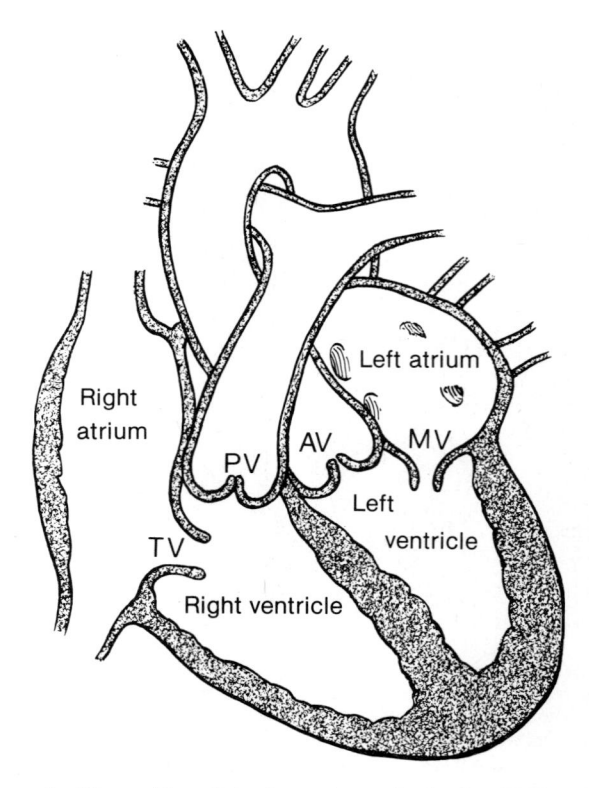

Figure 9 The position of the four valves: mitral valve (MV), aortic valve (AV), pulmonary valve (PV) and tricuspid valve (TV).

The Structure and Function of the Heart

Any blood tending to flow backwards pushes them shut. Figure 10 shows the details of these movements for the left side of the heart. The left ventricle draws blood into it by expanding, and opens the mitral valve lying between it and the left atrium (Figure 10a). At the same time the aortic valve closes. When the left ventricle contracts (Figure 10b), it squeezes blood out through the aortic valve, and the mitral valve connecting the ventricle and the atrium is pushed shut.

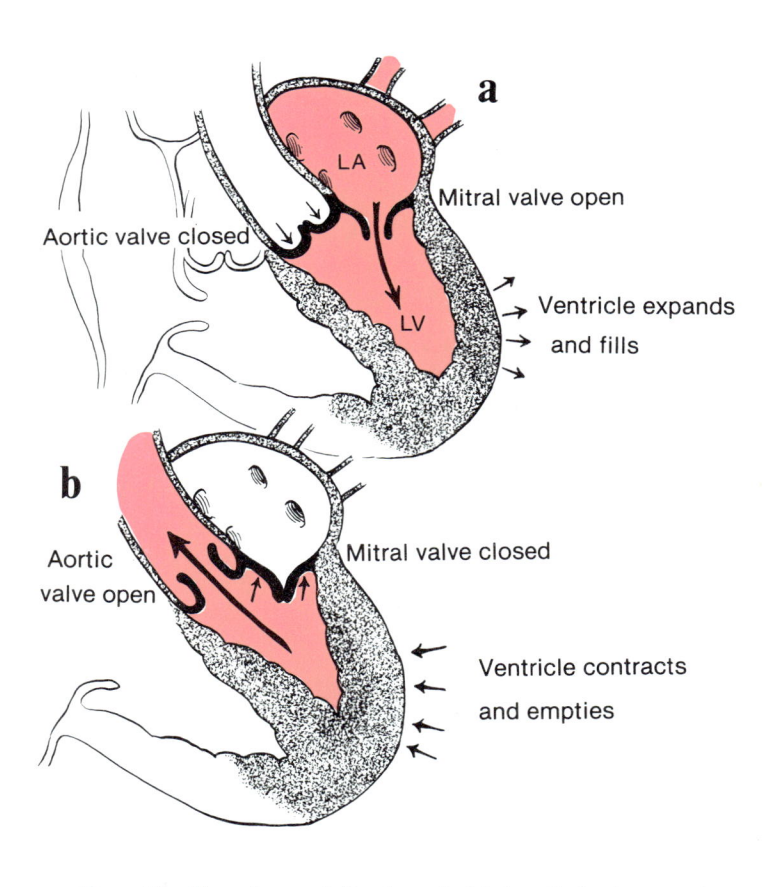

Figure 10 The valves work like doors. In (a) the mitral valve opens to allow the ventricle to fill. In (b) the mitral valve closes, and the aortic valve opens, as the ventricle pushes the blood out into the aorta.

11

Surgery and Your Heart

The Arteries of the Heart (Coronary Arteries)

The heart contracts 40–60 million times a year, working without a rest throughout our lives. In order to carry out this tremendous amount of work, it is important that the muscles of the heart are continuously supplied with oxygenated blood.

The oxygenated blood supply for the heart is supplied through two arteries, which branch off from the aorta immediately after it leaves the heart (Figure 11). These are the right and left coronary arteries, and they sub-divide into small branches which encircle the heart. It is from these coronary arteries that the heart muscle receives the oxygen it requires.

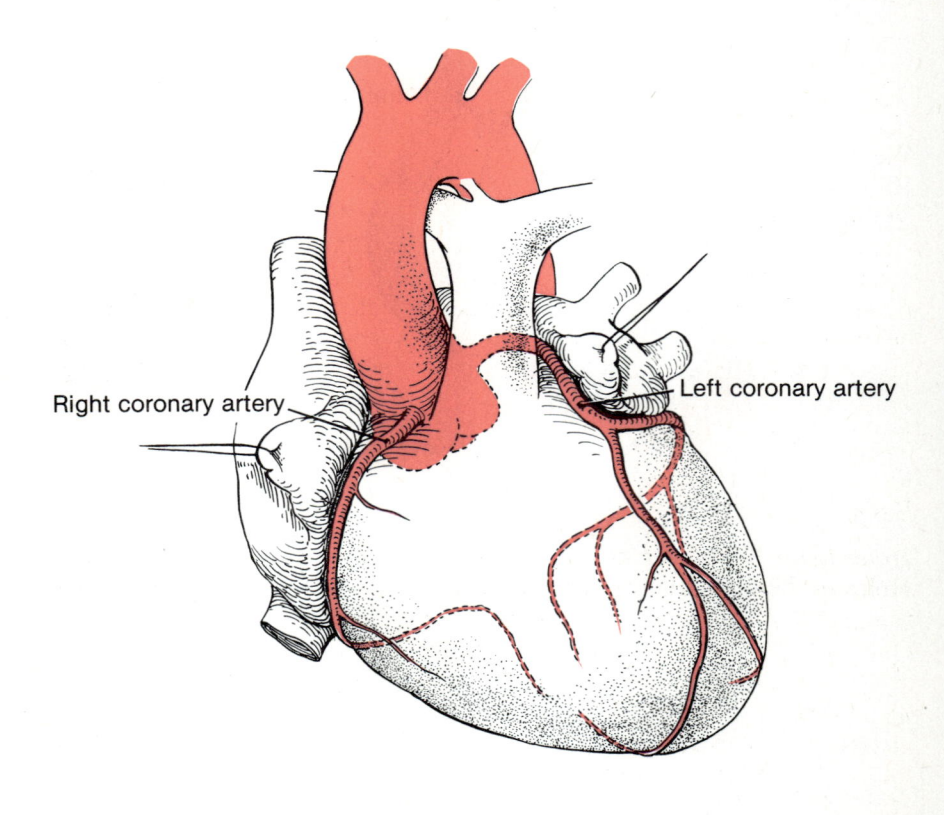

Figure 11 The outside of the heart, showing the course of the right and left coronary arteries.

Chapter 2
Diseases of the Heart

Diseases of the heart occur both before birth, while the heart is being formed in the foetus, and after birth. Diseases that occur while the heart is developing are called 'congenital diseases'. Those diseases that occur after birth are called 'acquired diseases' and are usually caused by gradual changes to the heart valves or the coronary arteries.

CONGENITAL HEART DISEASE

We will now look at some of the commoner conditions that arise before birth and which may cause problems to the newborn infant. Some of the simpler conditions consist of holes in the septa (walls between the heart chambers), a narrowing in the valves or major arteries, or abnormal connections between the large arteries.

There are more complicated disorders which combine several of these conditions. Some of the more serious conditions are the result of an abnormal circulation pattern being formed when the heart is developing, so that the chambers become connected to the wrong blood vessels or even fail to connect at all.

Simple Defects

Holes in the Septa: Atrial Septal Defect and Ventricular Septal Defect
Holes in the septa allow the red oxygenated blood and blue venous blood to mix. Such holes are among the most common congenital defects.

Atrial Septal Defect   When a hole occurs between the two low-pressure upper chambers (the atria), it is called an atrial septal defect. These holes can occur in different locations in the wall which normally divides the atria, but the effect in each case is to allow the red blood to mix with the blue (Figure 12a).

Atrial septal defects are easily repaired. The condition is commoner in

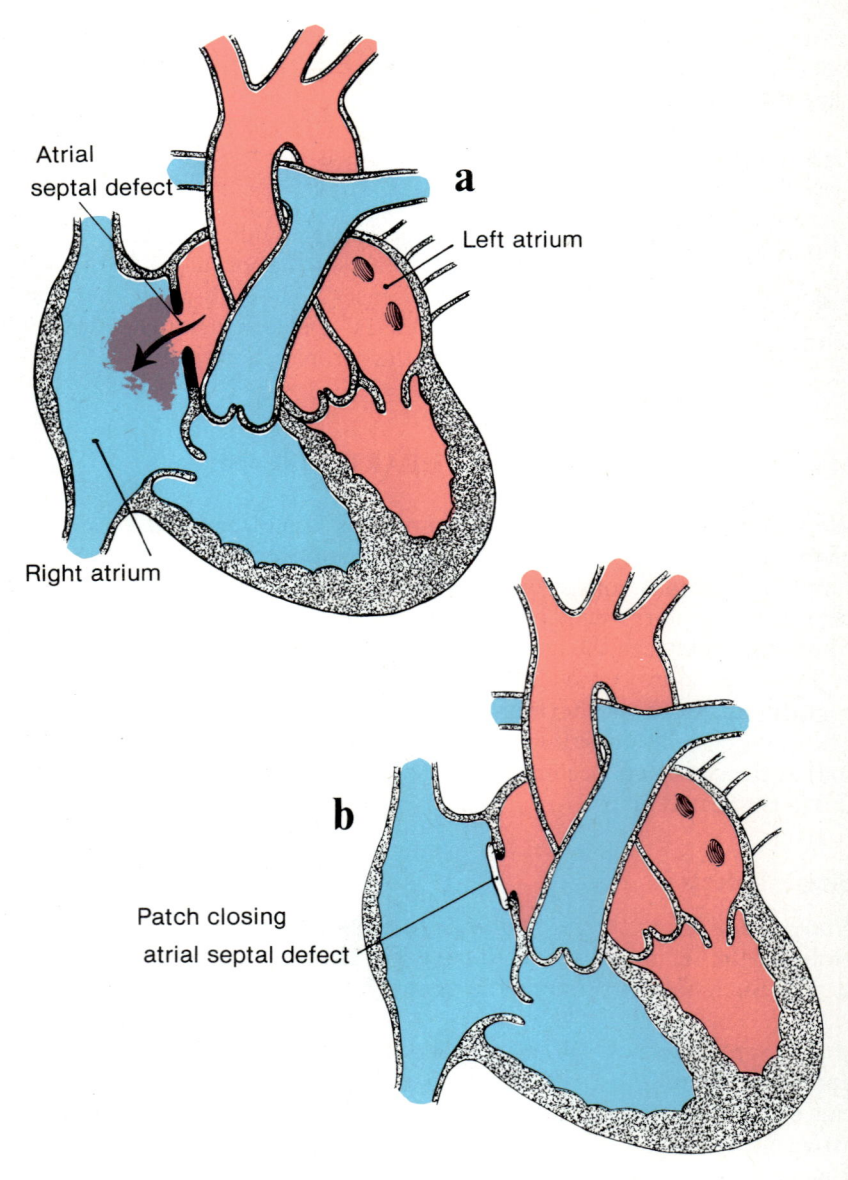

Figure 12   In (a) an atrial septal defect allows red blood from the left atrium to mix with the blue blood in the right atrium. In (b) the atrial septal defect has been closed with a patch sewn over the hole.

Diseases of the Heart

women and generally does not give rise to important symptoms till middle age. The hole can simply be sewn up, or it can be patched with a piece of surgical material (Figure 12b).

Ventricular Septal Defect   A hole in the septum separating the thick-walled ventricles is called a ventricular septal defect (Figure 13). This is a more important defect than an atrial septal defect, because of the high pressures that exist in these pumping chambers, and it is likely to give rise to symptoms at an early age or in infancy. However, just like the atrial septal defect, the ventricular septal defect is repaired by closing the hole with a patch.

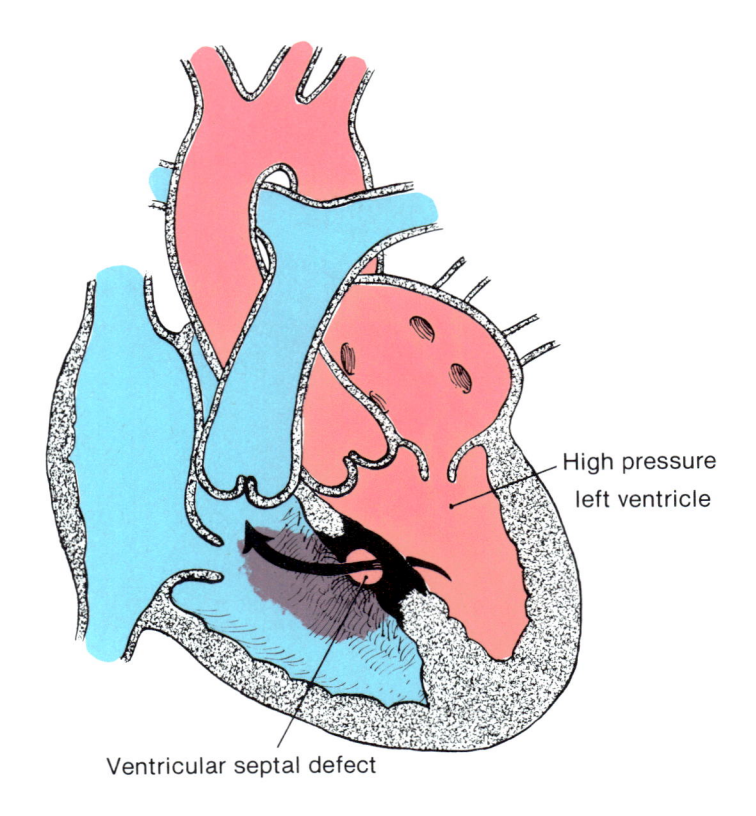

Figure 13 A ventricular septal defect is more important than an atrial septal defect because of the high pressures in the ventricles.

Narrowing of the Arteries: Pulmonary Stenosis and Coarctation of the Aorta

A narrowing in a blood vessel is called a stenosis. A fairly common congenital defect is to have a stenosis involving the blood vessel which carries blood from the right ventricle to the lungs. This is called pulmonary stenosis. When a narrowing occurs in the arch of the aorta it is called a coarctation of the aorta.

Pulmonary Stenosis Pulmonary stenosis can be a narrowing in the pulmonary artery itself, or below the valve, but is usually in the valve which allows blood to enter this artery (Figure 14). In either case, not enough blood gets through the narrowing on its way to the lungs to be oxygenated, and the body suffers from a lack of oxygen.

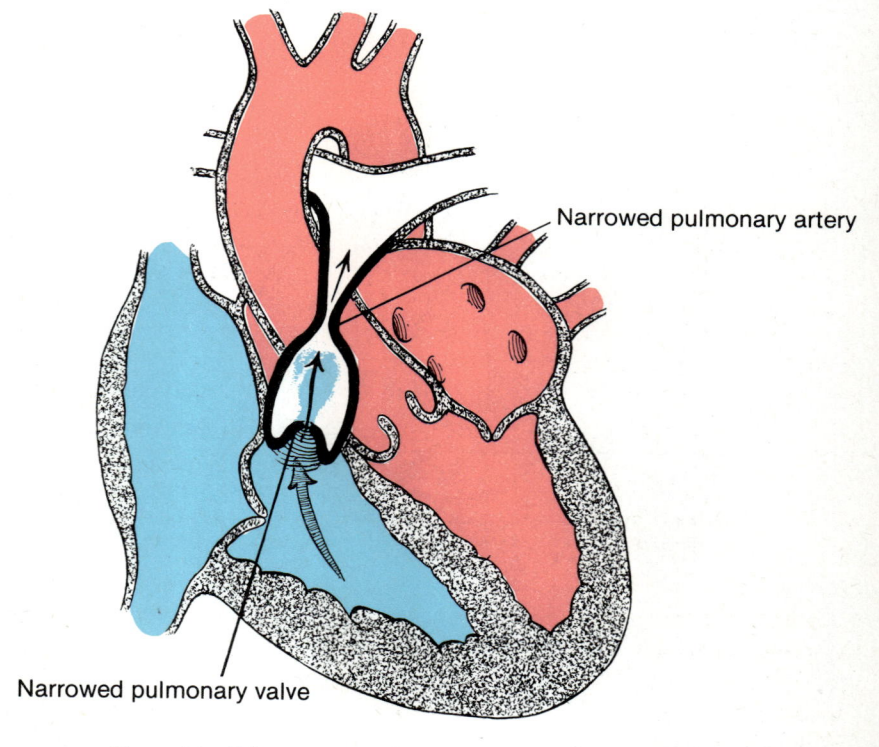

Figure 14 Pulmonary stenosis, showing both the common type of valve stenosis or narrowing, and how the pulmonary artery itself may be the cause of the obstruction.

Diseases of the Heart

This defect is simply treated by opening the valve or enlarging the narrow area. In more complicated cases, a new bypass channel can be made between the right ventricle and the pulmonary artery beyond the narrowing or obstruction (Figure 15).

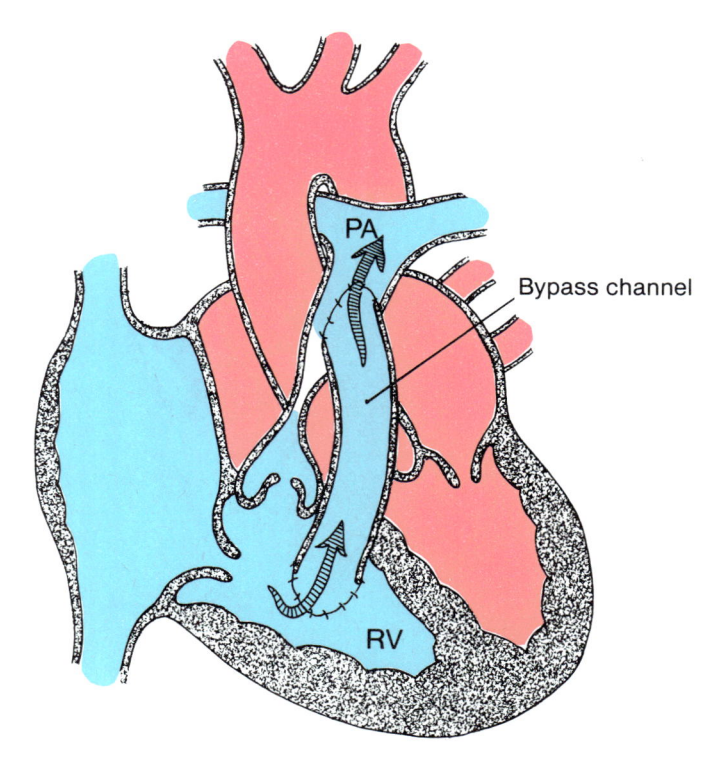

Figure 15 A bypass channel has been sewn in place so that blood from the right ventricle can flow freely around the narrowed valve or artery.

Coarctation of the Aorta When a narrowing occurs in the aorta beyond the point at which it gives off its branches to the head, it is called a coarctation of the aorta. Small bridging arteries (Figure 16a) develop, which carry blood around the coarctation. In this way, the legs and organs receive their blood but pressure builds up in the aorta in front of the obstruction.

Surgery and Your Heart

The two most common ways of correcting a coarctation are shown in Figures 16b and 16c. In (b) the surgeon has removed the narrowed segment and has sewn the two cut ends together. In (c) a patch has been sewn into the aorta, which widens the narrowed part. The result of both operations is that the blood can flow freely to the lower part of the body and the pressure in the aorta and head vessels is relieved.

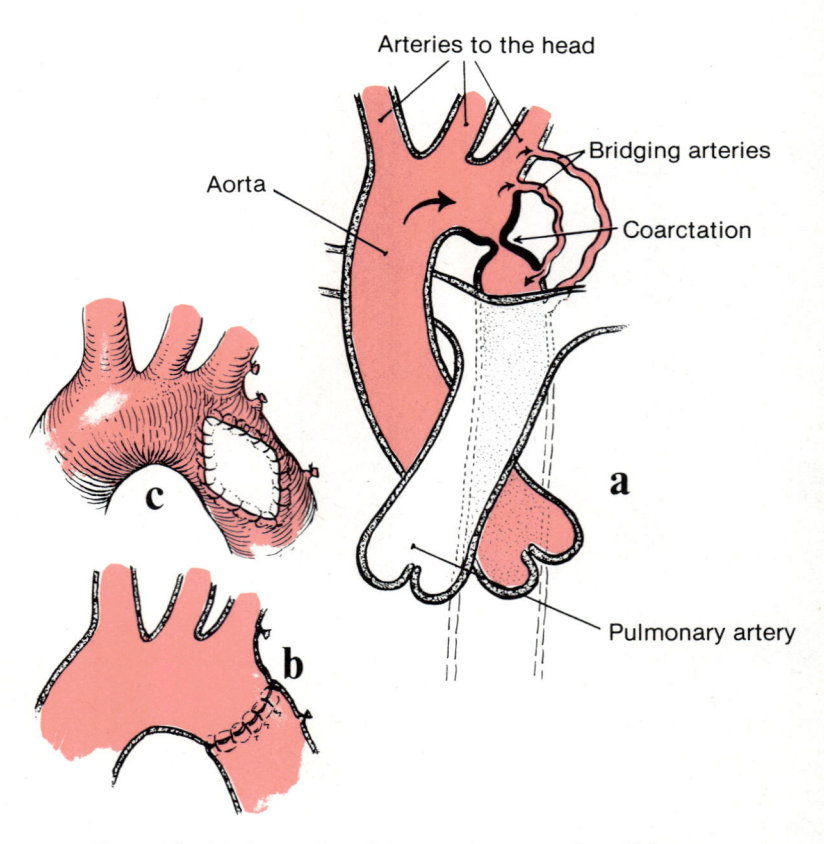

Figure 16 (a) Coarctation of the aorta is a narrowing which occurs just beyond the arteries to the head. Blood flows around the narrowing in small bridging arteries. (b) The narrowed segment has been removed and the two ends of the aorta have been sewn together. (c) A patch can be used to widen the narrow area.

18

Diseases of the Heart

Abnormal Connections: Patent Ductus Arteriosus
The ductus arteriosus is a short artery which connects the aorta to the pulmonary artery. Before the infant's birth, this artery is open and carries blood from the pulmonary artery to the aorta (bypassing the non-functioning lungs). Soon after birth, the ductus arteriosus closes. In some cases, however, it fails to close and remains 'patent' (open) (Figure 17a). This causes the red blood in the aorta to mix with the blue blood in the pulmonary artery, and the lungs are filled with an excessive amount of

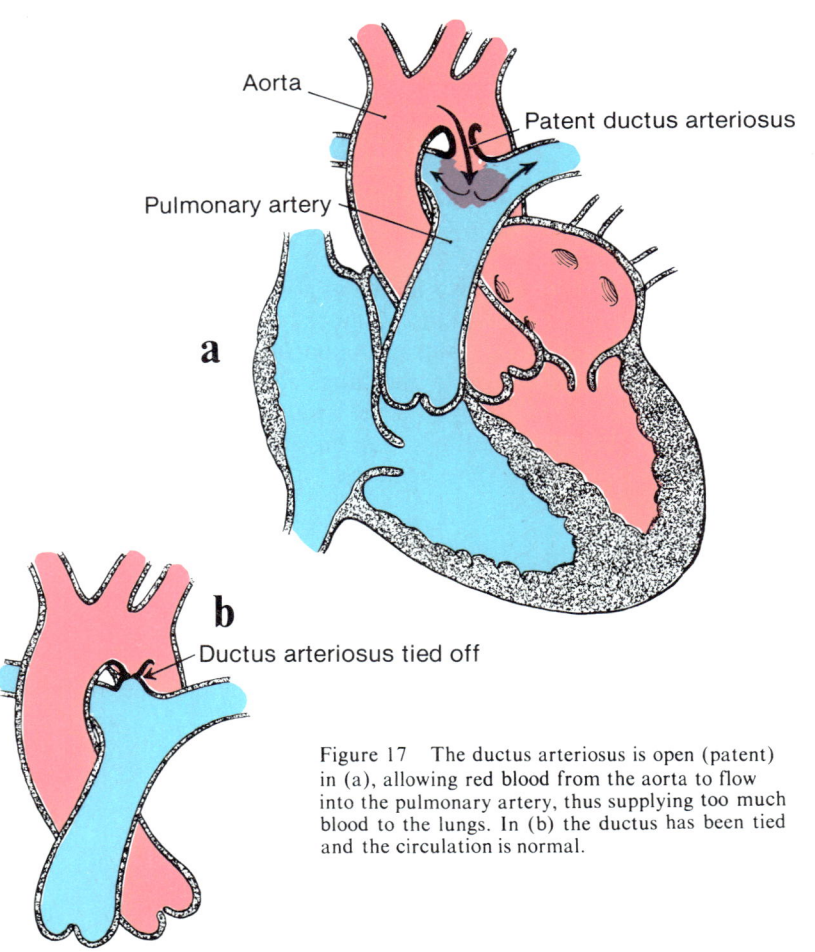

Figure 17 The ductus arteriosus is open (patent) in (a), allowing red blood from the aorta to flow into the pulmonary artery, thus supplying too much blood to the lungs. In (b) the ductus has been tied and the circulation is normal.

blood at an increased pressure. The lungs become stiff and breathing is difficult.

Surgeons can treat this condition by tying off or dividing the ductus arteriosus (Figure 17b). This was one of the earliest heart operations carried out.

Complex Defects

Tetralogy of Fallot
This condition includes several of the already discussed simple abnormalities. It is one of a few diseases which cause the baby's skin to have a bluish colouring, known by the medical term 'cyanosis'. It is the result of a mixture of blue and red blood being distributed to the tissues.

Babies born with a tetralogy of Fallot are blue and breathless. They develop more slowly than normal children and are breathless on mild exertion. When they are older, they squat on their heels when they are tired.

In this condition there are two major abnormalities (Figure 18). The first is a narrowing or stenosis of the pulmonary artery (see page 16). This makes the child breathless, tired and poorly developed, because not enough blood gets oxygenated in the lungs for the nourishment of the tissues. The second abnormality is a ventricular septal defect (see page 15). This hole in the septum allows blue blood from the obstructed right ventricle to escape into the left ventricle. It then flows to the tissues, making the child's skin blue.

Diseases of the Heart

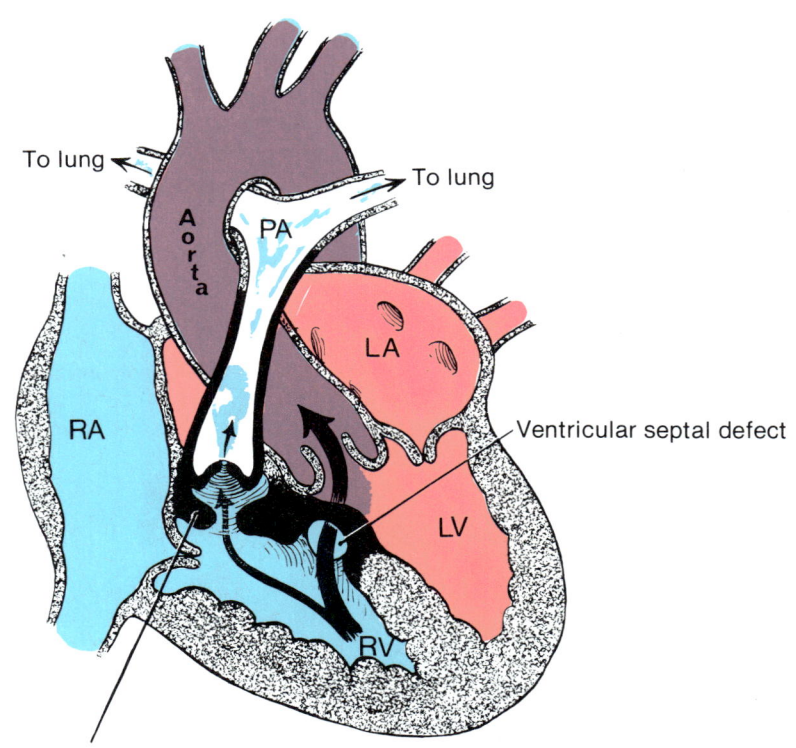

Figure 18 Diagram to show the two main abnormalities in Fallot's tetralogy: 1) pulmonary stenosis, which obstructs the flow of blood to the lungs, and 2) a ventricular septal defect, which allows the blue blood to mix with the red. This gives the skin its purplish colour (cyanosis).

Surgery and Your Heart

There are several ways of treating the tetralogy of Fallot. One way is to create a passageway between the aorta and pulmonary artery so that more blood can flow to the lungs to pick up oxygen (Figure 19). There are different ways of creating this passageway. In Figure 19, an artery which normally goes to the left arm is joined to the pulmonary artery. This operation, called the Blalock shunt operation, improves the child's condition dramatically because more blood now reaches the lungs to be oxygenated. The shunt operation is usually done in very young babies, and further surgery is required when the child is older.

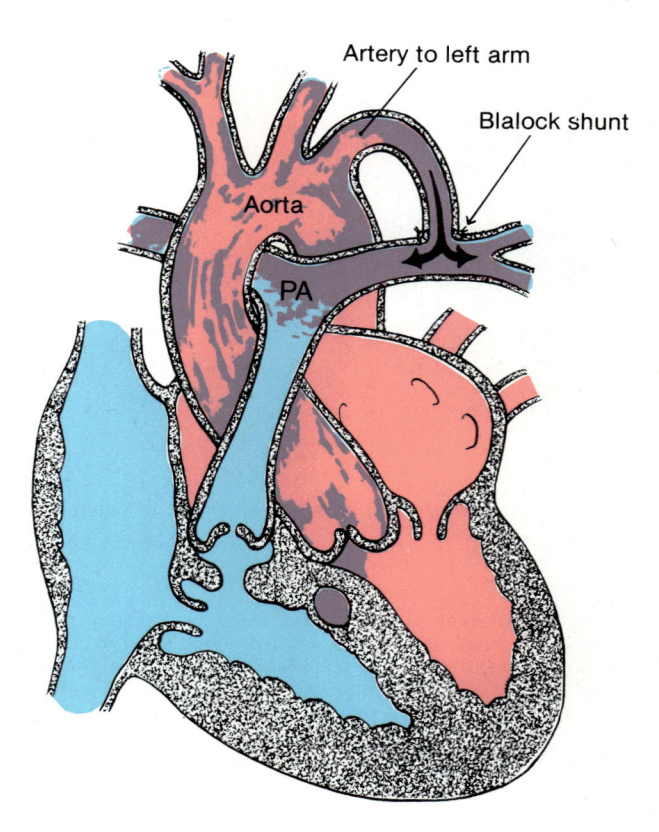

Figure 19 The Blalock shunt is created by joining the artery which normally goes to the left arm to the left pulmonary artery, so that more blood can flow to the lungs to become oxygenated. The left arm circulation is not at risk.

Diseases of the Heart

The ideal way to treat this condition is to do a complete or total correction of a tetralogy of Fallot (Figure 20). The surgeon opens the heart and removes the pulmonary stenosis or obstruction to the flow of blood to the lungs. He then sews a patch over the ventricular septal defect, which stops the blue and red blood from mixing. If there had been an earlier shunt operation, the connection is tied off or disconnected. The result is that all the blue blood flows through the lungs and emerges as red blood to supply the tissues.

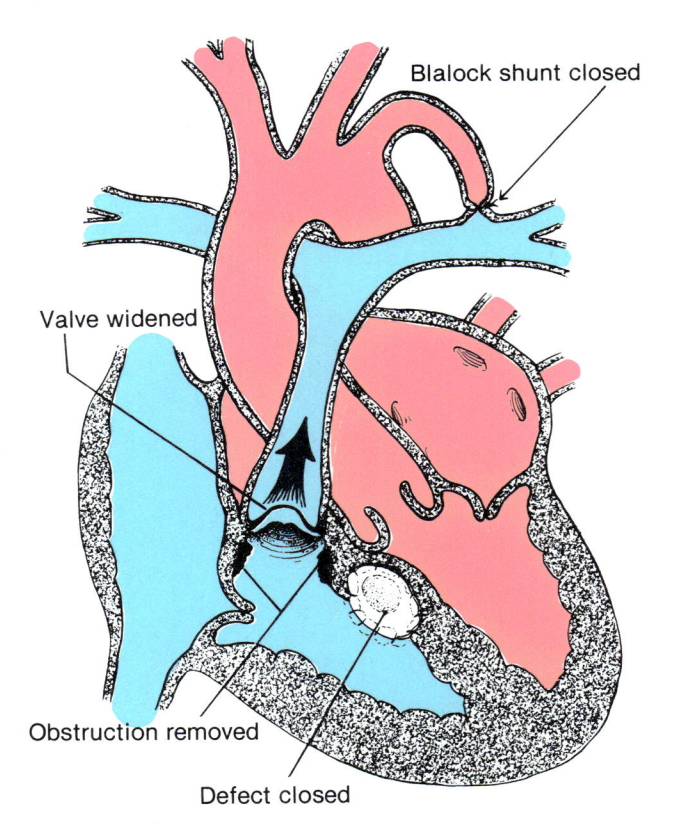

Figure 20   The total correction of the tetralogy of Fallot. In this diagram the valve stenosis has been removed by widening the valve opening, the muscular obstruction below the valve has been removed and the ventricular septal defect has been closed with a patch. Also the previous Blalock shunt from Figure 19 has been closed.

Surgery and Your Heart

Transposition of the Great Arteries
Transposition is another disease that causes severe 'cyanosis', particularly in newborn infants. These blue babies often die within a few hours or days after birth if they are not treated.

The term 'transposition of the great arteries' means that the main arteries which leave the heart – the aorta and the pulmonary artery – are transposed, or connected to the wrong ventricles. Because of this, blue blood from the tissues enters the right atrium, passes into the right ventricle, and is pumped out to the organs and body tissues through the aorta instead of to the lungs. Red blood from the lungs enters the left atrium and left ventricle and is pumped back to the lungs again, via the wrongly-connected pulmonary artery. If the red and blue circuits are unable to mix through holes or communications in the heart, the infant will not live more than a few minutes. Usually, however, there is an atrial septal defect, ventricular septal defect, patent ductus arteriosus, or several of these communications, allowing some blue and red blood to mix together and maintain a precarious existence for the baby (Figure 21).

Diseases of the Heart

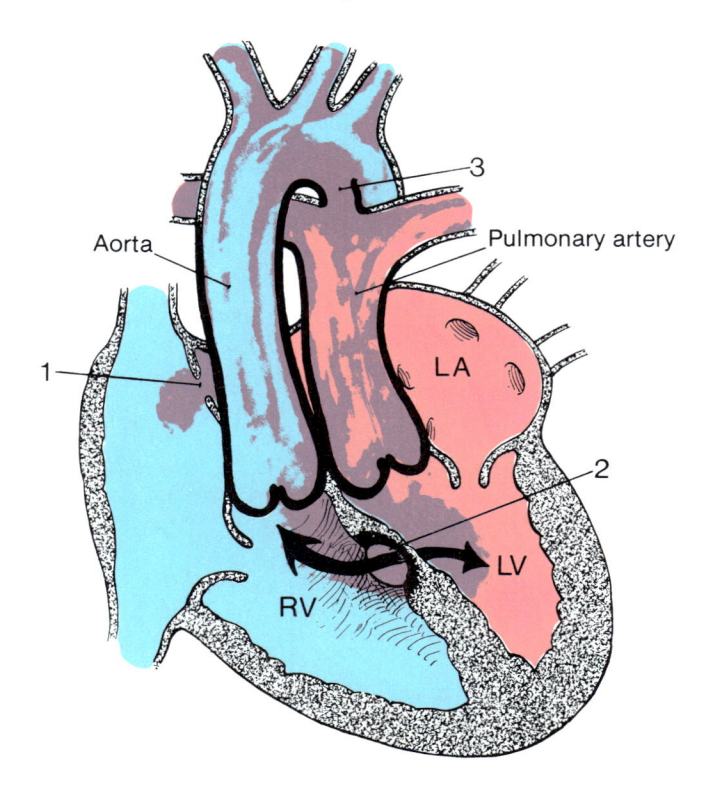

Figure 21 Diagram of a heart with transposition of the great arteries, showing the incorrect connection of the aorta to the right ventricle and the pulmonary artery to the left ventricle. Also shown are three possible communications between the right and left sides of the heart which may keep the baby alive by allowing red and blue blood to mix: 1) an atrial septal defect, 2) a ventricular septal defect and 3) a patent ductus arteriosus.

If the condition is diagnosed early enough, the baby can be improved quickly. The cardiologist makes a large hole in the septum between the atria (Figure 22), by threading a deflated little balloon attached to the end of a thin tube into the right atrium by way of a vein. The balloon and tube are threaded through the atrial wall into the left atrium. The balloon is then inflated and pulled back forcibly through the septum, creating a large hole that allows red blood from the lungs to flow freely into the right side of the heart. This improves the baby's condition dramatically, by allowing some oxygenated blood to pass to the tissues.

Surgery and Your Heart

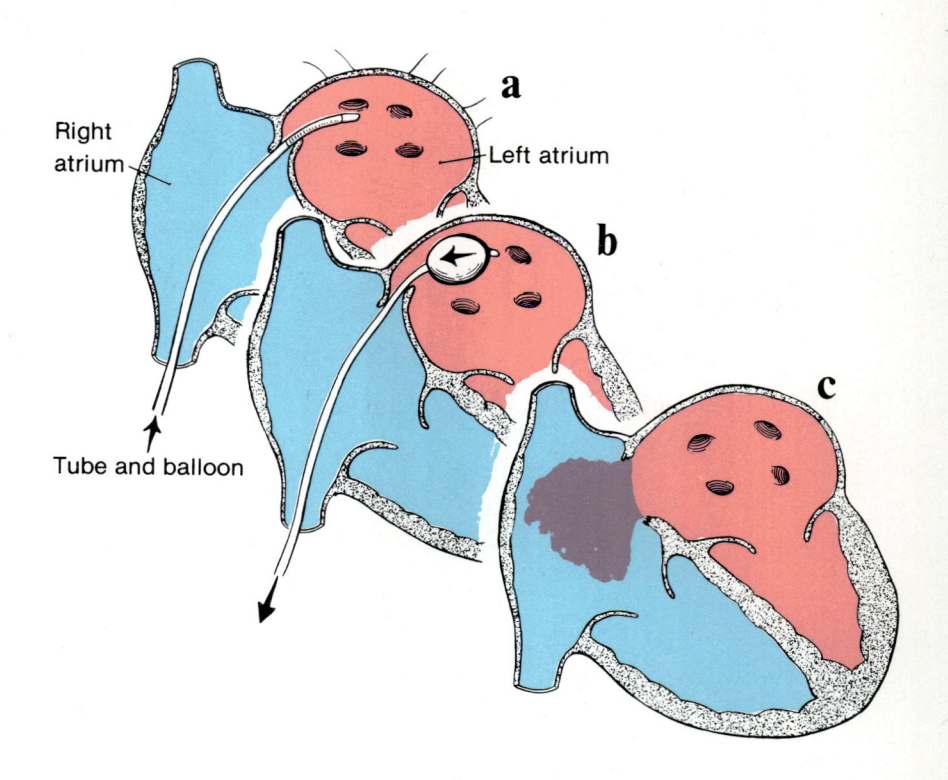

Figure 22 This Rashkind procedure will improve the baby's condition dramatically. The instrument used is a thin tube with a balloon attached to its end. The balloon can be inflated once it is in place. In (a) the balloon has been threaded into the heart through a vein and has been pushed into the left atrium. In (b) the balloon is inflated and is pulled back forcibly into the right atrium, thereby creating a large hole in the atrial septum. In (c) the tube has been removed, and the hole now allows a large amount of red blood to mix with the blue.

When older, the child can be treated surgically by rearranging the existing pattern of the two circulations. This is achieved by redirecting (1) the blue blood to the lungs, and (2) the red blood to the aorta and body. There are two ways to accomplish this. The commonest operation is called the Mustard operation, which corrects the transposition by changing the pattern of circulation entering the pumping chambers, or ventricles (Figure 23).

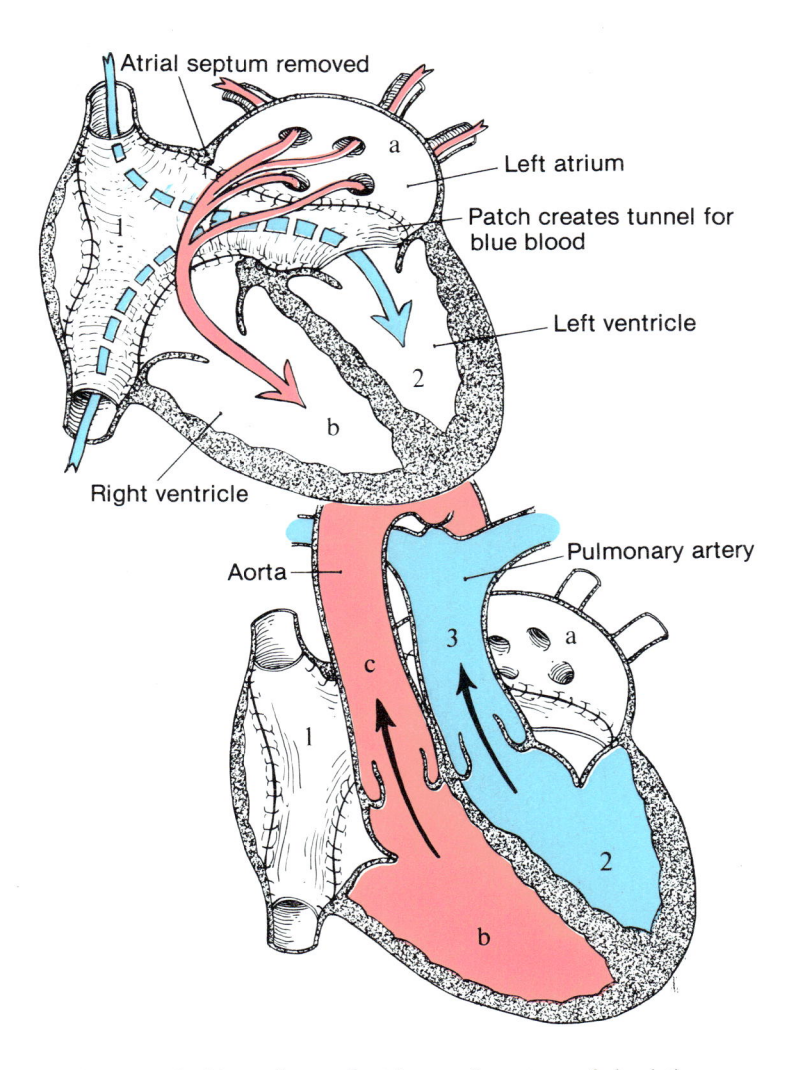

Figure 23 The Mustard operation changes the pattern of circulation entering the ventricles. In the upper diagram the atrial septum has been removed by the surgeon, creating one chamber out of the two atria. A large patch is then sewn into this chamber in such a way as to create a tunnel (1), through which the blue blood coming from the body is redirected through the mitral valve and into the left ventricle (2). The red blood from the lungs flows over the new tunnel (a) and through the tricuspid valve into the right ventricle (b). In the lower diagram the red blood is now pumped out of the heart through the aorta (c) and flows to the tissues. The blue blood now flows to the lungs via the pulmonary artery (3), as in the normal circulation.

Surgery and Your Heart

The alternative operation is called the switch operation. The aorta and the pulmonary artery are simply cut across, switched to their correct sides and restitched (Figure 24). In this way, the blue blood now flows out of the heart to the lungs, via the switched-over pulmonary artery, and red blood leaves the heart via the aorta as in the normal heart.

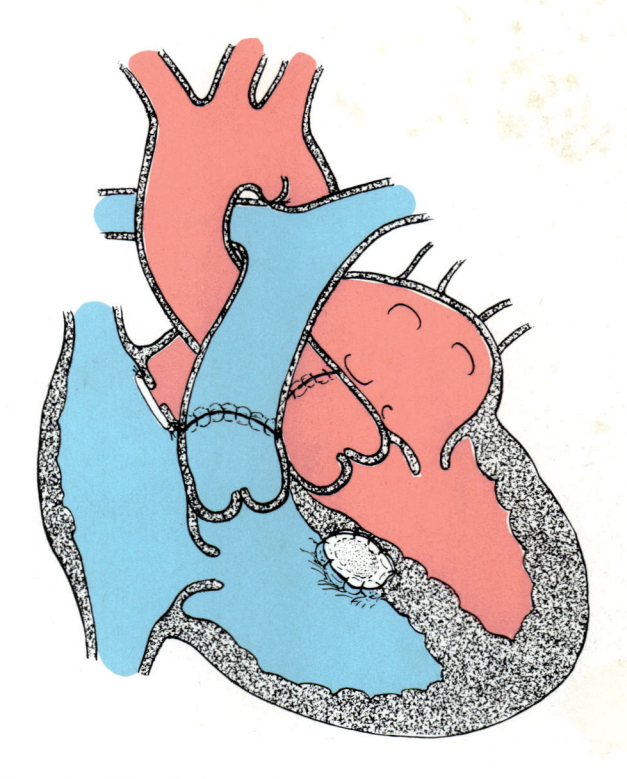

Figure 24   The switch operation. Both major arteries have been cut across near the heart and switched to their correct sides. The three communications from Figure 21 have been closed.

There are several other conditions that are less common than those discussed. Many operations have been developed to treat congenital heart abnormalities, so that there are now very few conditions which cannot be helped in some way by means of surgery.

Diseases of the Heart

ACQUIRED DISEASES OF THE HEART

Coronary Heart Disease and Heart Attacks

As we have seen in the introductory chapter, the coronary arteries encircle the heart (Figure 25) and provide it with a constant supply of oxy-

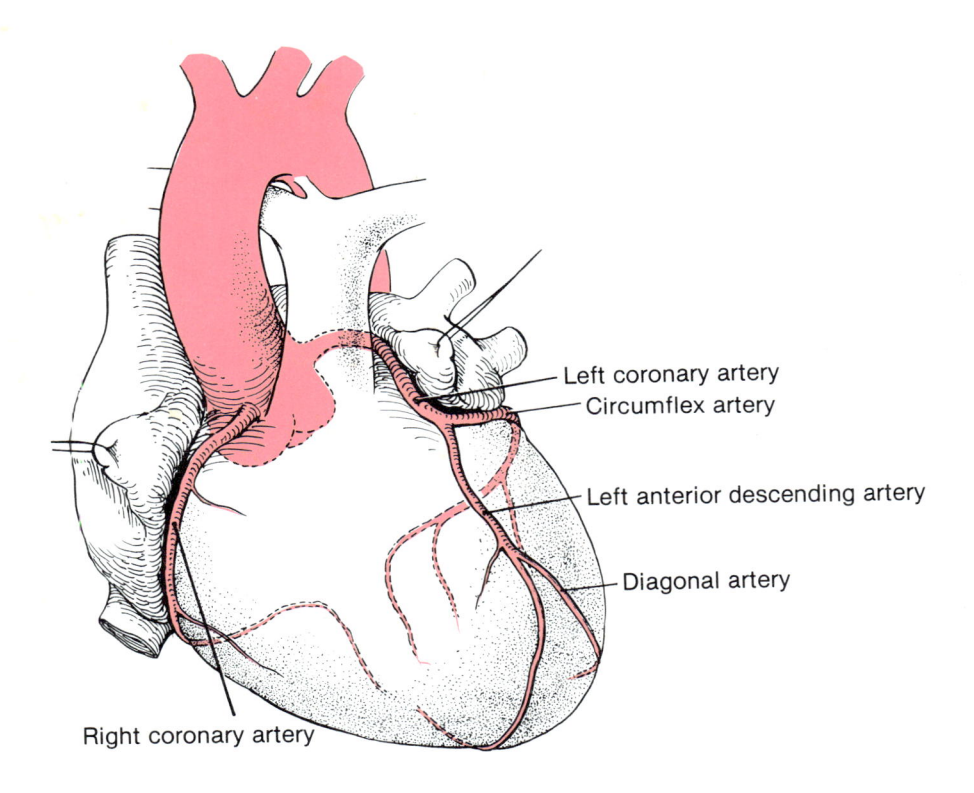

Figure 25 Diagram of the heart showing the two main coronary arteries (the right and left coronary arteries) and their main branches. The left main coronary artery originates from the aorta, going behind the pulmonary artery before it appears on the front of the heart. It branches, and one of its branches (the circumflex artery) follows the groove between the left atrium and left ventricle around to the back of the heart. The other branch (the left anterior descending artery) follows the groove between the right and left ventricles down the front of the heart. The right main coronary artery runs down the groove between the right atrium and right ventricle and follows it around to the back of the heart.

Surgery and Your Heart

genated blood. This supplies the energy to maintain its pumping action. Any interference with the flow of blood in the coronary arteries will have a serious effect on the heart muscle and its ability to pump the blood out to the head, neck, arms, legs and organs.

Angina
At certain sites in the course of the coronary arteries, fatty substances may slowly build up on the inner walls of the arteries. These deposits gradually narrow the lumen of the arteries (space available for blood in the vessel) and restrict the blood flow to the heart muscle, giving rise to pain (Figure 26).

This patient will probably first experience angina when his heart is beating faster, such as when he is exercising or feeling emotionally upset. Angina is a pain felt in the central chest and perhaps in the neck and arms. It means that not enough blood is reaching the heart muscle through the narrowed arteries. The pain does not last long and usually stops when the heart slows down, when the exercise or emotional disturbance is over, or when the patient puts an appropriate pill under his tongue.

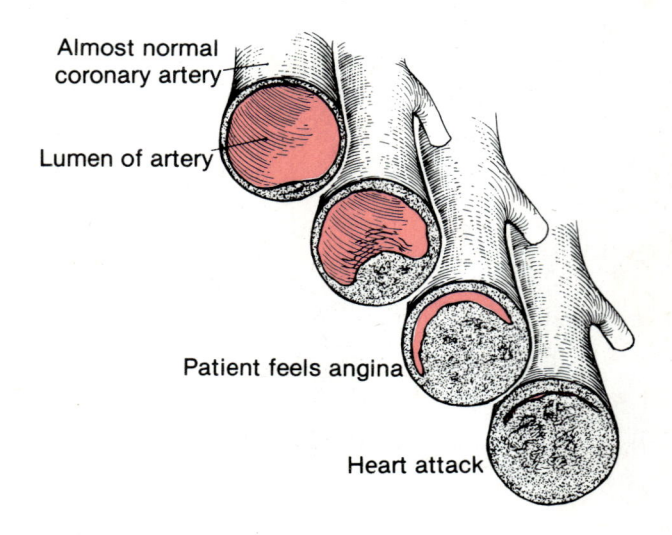

Figure 26 Diagram showing the cross section of an artery with progressive build-up of fatty substances which eventually block the inside of the artery. This diagram shows the same artery probably over a period of years.

Diseases of the Heart

Angina can be treated with pills which dilate the smaller arteries or reduce the amount of oxygen that the heart needs. More often these days a coronary artery bypass operation is carried out.

In the coronary artery bypass operation, the surgeon removes a long segment of vein from the patient's leg and uses this vein to form a new pathway for the blood to get to the muscle. One end of the vein is sewn to the aorta, and the other end to the diseased coronary artery beyond the blockage (Figure 27). This 'vein graft' bypasses the obstruction and brings in a new supply of blood to the deprived heart muscle. Figure 27 illustrates a blockage or narrowing in two coronary arteries, and the vein grafts used to bypass the obstructions.

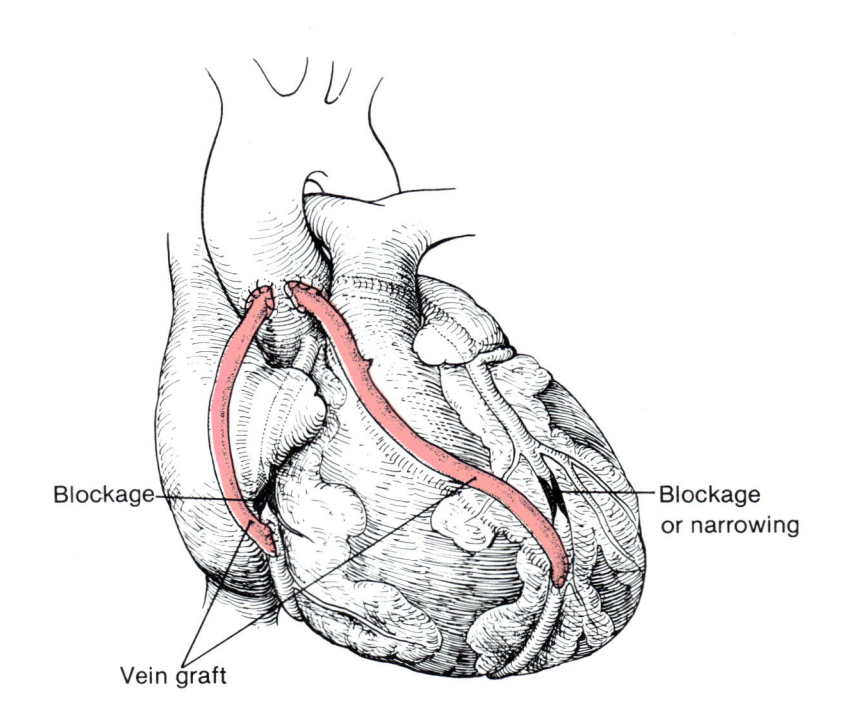

Figure 27   Drawing of the heart with two vein grafts sewn into place to bypass two narrowed arteries. Blood leaving the heart from the aorta will flow into the vein grafts and bring oxygen to the heart muscle beyond the blockages.

Surgery and Your Heart

Heart Attack
A sudden blockage may occur in one of the narrowed coronary arteries. This prevents blood from reaching the heart muscle supplied by that artery (Figure 28). A blockage like this is commonly called a 'heart attack'. It may also be called 'coronary thrombosis' or 'myocardial infarction'. The person having such a heart attack experiences a severe prolonged pain in the chest, or may actually die.

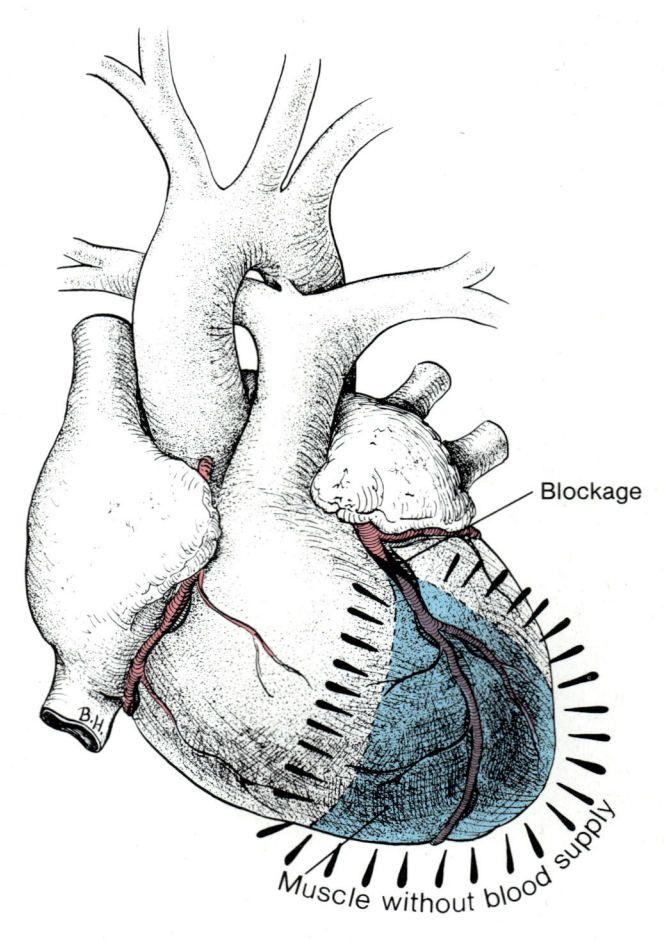

Figure 28 This diagram shows that a triangular area of heart muscle beyond a blockage will suffer from a lack of oxygen, with consequent damage to that area of the heart muscle.

Diseases of the Heart

After he recovers from a heart attack, the patient may feel perfectly well, or may have anginal pain or breathlessness. The symptoms depend upon the amount of heart muscle which has been damaged by the lack of oxygen, and also upon the amount of disease in the remaining coronary arteries. If the heart muscle is not badly damaged but the coronary arteries are narrow, the patient will have angina upon exertion or emotional stress, or possibly even while sleeping.

In other patients, the heart attack may permanently damage a part of the heart muscle so that it can no longer contract effectively. Repeated heart attacks damage more and more heart muscle, leaving the patient with a large, unhealthy and poorly contracting heart (Figure 29). When such a heart contracts, insufficient blood is pumped to the body, making breathlessness the predominant symptom. At this stage in the disease, not a great deal can be done with surgery. The aim of medical management of the patient with coronary artery disease should be to prevent this sort of damage, which is usually the end result of a number of repeated heart attacks.

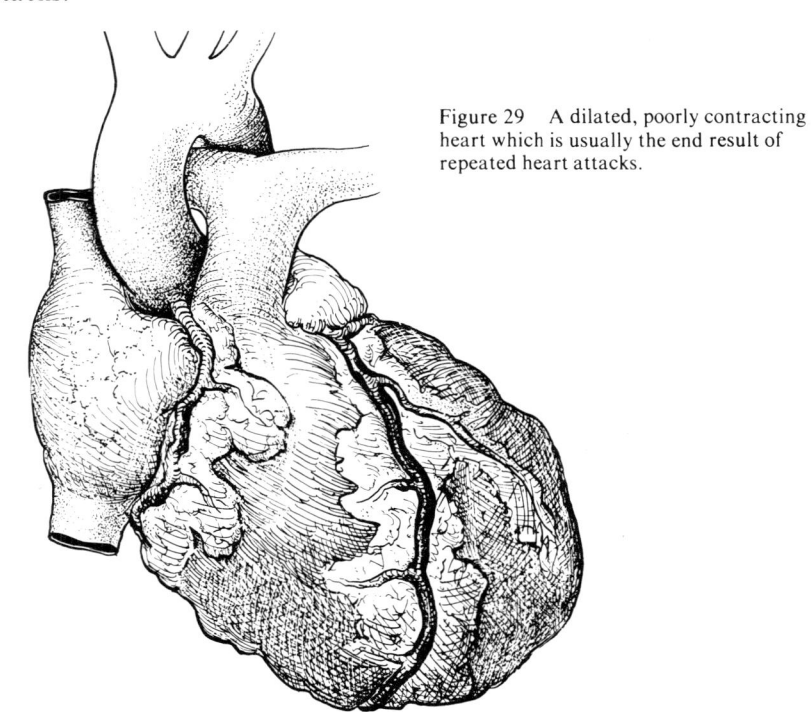

Figure 29 A dilated, poorly contracting heart which is usually the end result of repeated heart attacks.

Surgery and Your Heart

Aneurysm

Sometimes a localised area of damaged heart muscle protrudes as a bulge (Figure 30). This is called an 'aneurysm'. These aneurysms often contain a clot which may fly off into the circulation. Also they represent an area of non-functioning heart wall which can add to the work of the heart. The surgeon can safely remove such an aneurysm from the ventricle at the same time as the bypass operation. This restores a more normal pumping action to the heart.

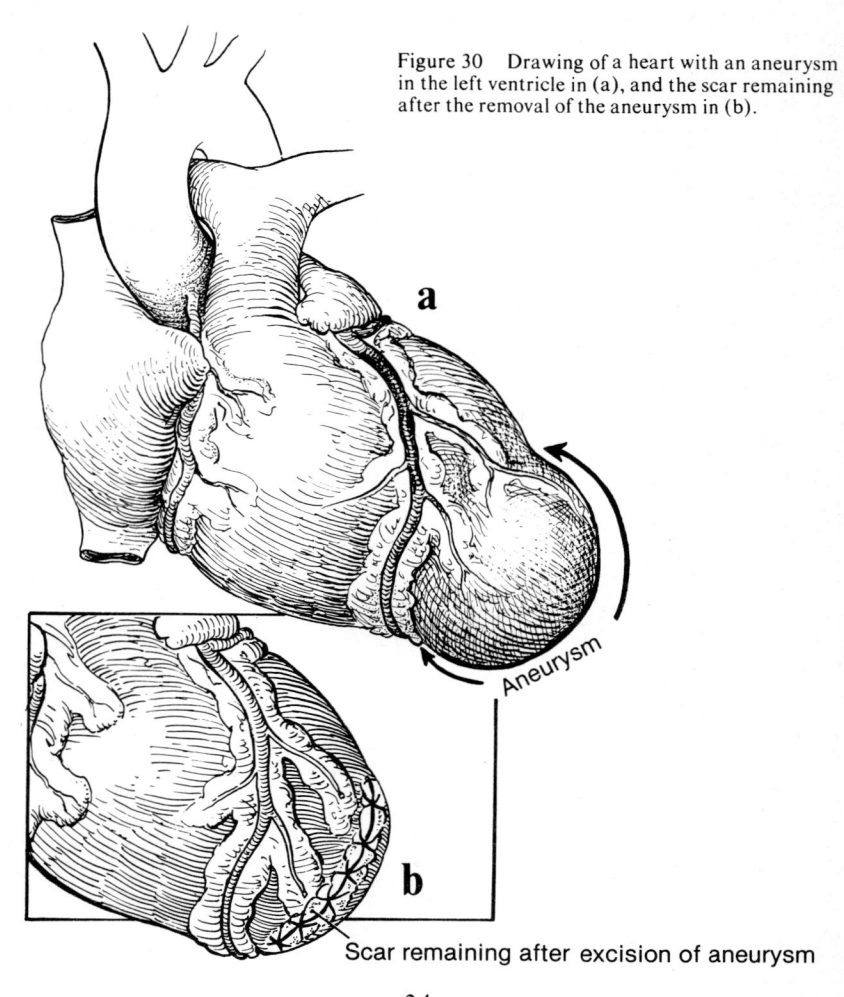

Figure 30 Drawing of a heart with an aneurysm in the left ventricle in (a), and the scar remaining after the removal of the aneurysm in (b).

Diseases of the Valves

Causes of Valve Disease

We have seen how the valves ensure that blood flows in only one direction in the heart (Figures 3, 9 and 10). There are several diseases which affect the valves' ability to open and close properly.

The commonest cause of valve disease is rheumatic fever. Rheumatic fever generally occurs in childhood following recurrent sore throats, and gives rise to fever and painful swelling of the joints of the arms and legs. This disease is common in countries surrounding the Mediterranean Sea, the Middle East and the Far East, or in conditions of overcrowding and poor nutrition.

When rheumatic fever affects the heart, it causes an inflammation of the valves. As they heal, the leaflets (or cusps) often stick together to form a narrowed valve (stenosis). The stenotic valve allows less blood to pass through the opening and the pressure of blood behind the obstruction builds up. Figures 31 and 32 show two aortic valves as seen from above. Figures 31a and 31b show a normal valve with thin leaflets in the closed and open positions. Figure 32 shows an aortic valve with stenosis, resulting from rheumatic fever. The leaflets are thickened and stuck together to leave a narrow opening. Figures 33 and 34 show the same views of the mitral valve before and after the rheumatic infection.

Surgery and Your Heart

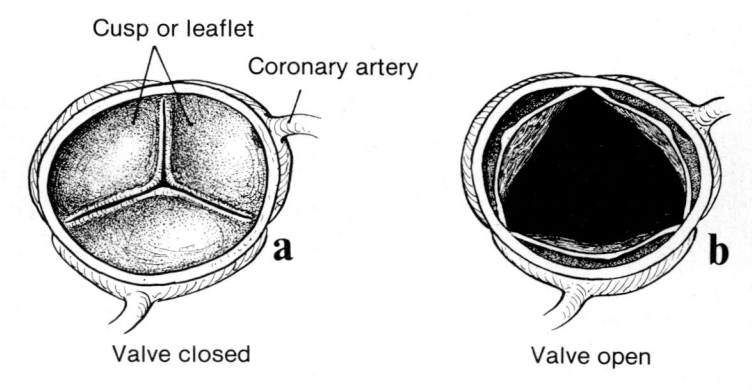

Figure 31 The surgeon's view of the normal aortic valve. In (a) the valve is closed to prevent blood from flowing back, and in (b) the valve is open to allow blood to escape from the ventricle.

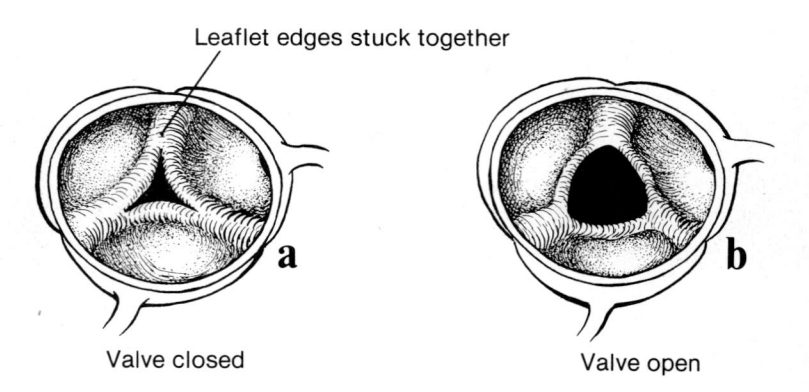

Figure 32 The same view of the aortic valve as Figure 31 (from above). This valve is stenotic as a result of rheumatic fever. The three cusps of the valve have fused together leaving a narrow central opening. Again, (a) is the closed position and (b) is the open position.

Diseases of the Heart

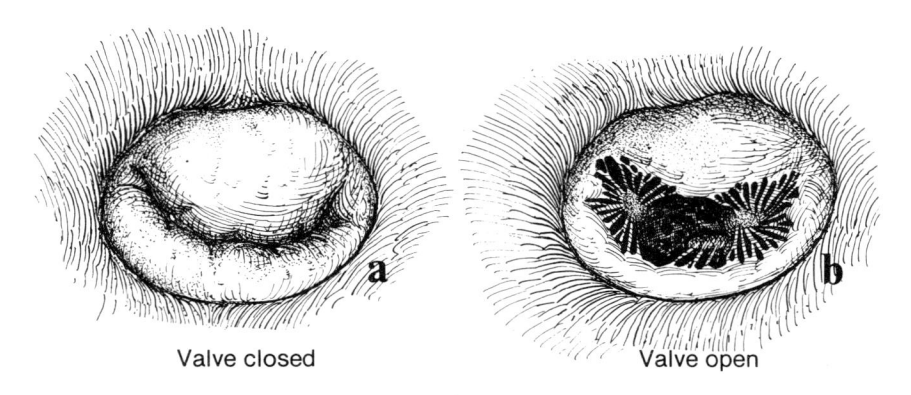

Valve closed   Valve open

Figure 33 The view of the normal mitral valve as seen from the left atrium. In (a) the mitral valve is closed, preventing blood from escaping from the left ventricle, and (b) is the open position, allowing blood to flow forwards from the lungs and left atrium.

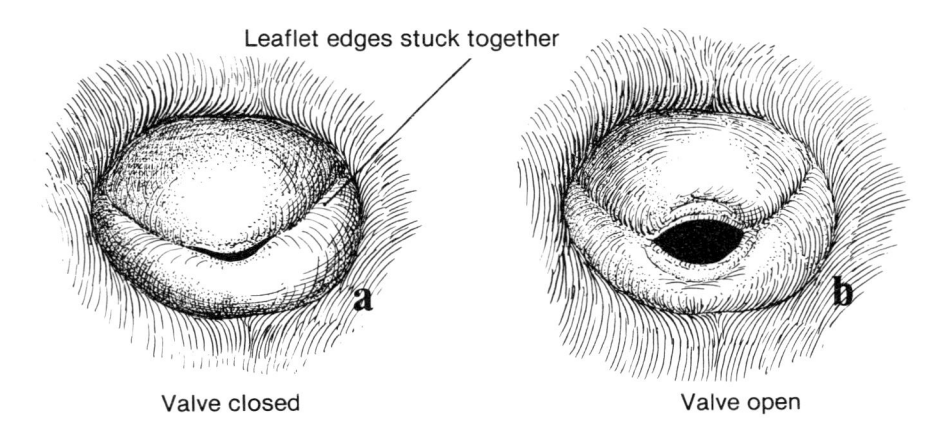

Leaflet edges stuck together

Valve closed   Valve open

Figure 34 The same view of the mitral valve as in Figure 33. This valve is stenotic as a result of rheumatic fever. The edges of the two cusps are fused together: (a) is the closed position and (b) is the open position.

Surgery and Your Heart

If the inflamed edges of the leaflets are thickened and shrink, the valve then cannot close and blood leaks backwards. This means that the heart has to work harder to pump enough blood to the body. They are called 'regurgitant' valves – Figure 35 shows a regurgitant aortic valve and Figure 36 a regurgitant mitral valve. 'Insufficiency' is another term for regurgitation.

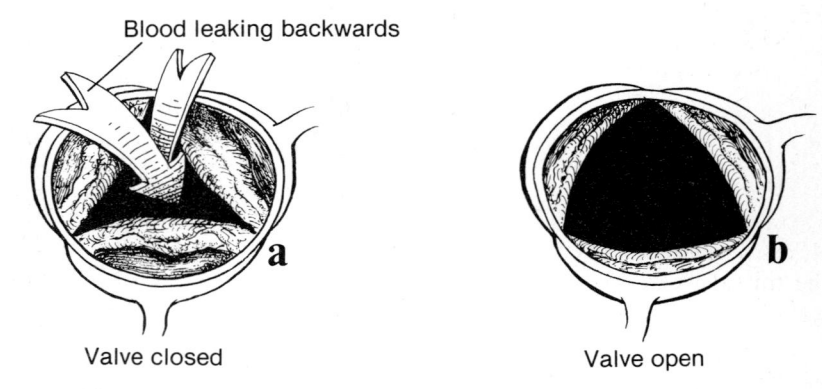

Figure 35 A regurgitant aortic valve in the closed (a) and open (b) positions. The cusps are damaged so that the valve cannot close, and blood flows backwards (arrowed) into the left ventricle.

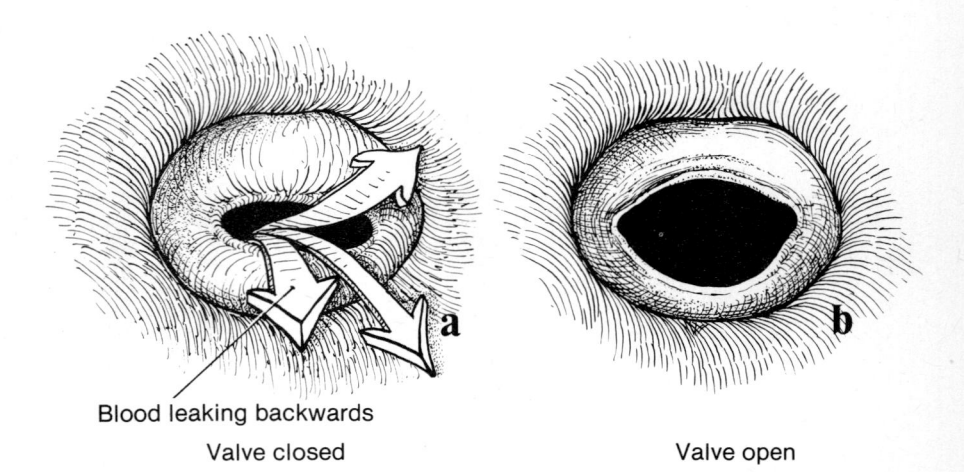

Figure 36 A regurgitant mitral valve, seen from above, in the closed (a) and open (b) positions. Blood leaks backwards (arrowed) into the left atrium.

Diseases of the Heart

In Western Europe and in the United States of America the commonest cause of valve disease is a congenital (inborn) irregularity of the aortic valve. In later life, this abnormal valve becomes covered by chalky deposits which make the valve rigid and unable to open or close properly. This is called calcific aortic stenosis and is shown in Figure 37.

Figure 37 The aortic valve resulting from congenital aortic stenosis. It is covered by chalky deposits and is rigid.

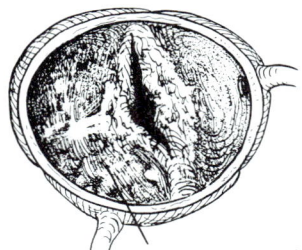

Chalky deposits

Stenosis of the Valves
Mitral Stenosis Mitral stenosis results from rheumatic fever affecting the mitral valve. As the inflamed valve heals, its leaflets stick together, leaving it with a small opening. Red oxygenated blood coming from the lungs is held up in its passage from the left atrium. Since blood is still being pumped freely into the lungs by the right ventricles, and cannot escape freely through the narrowed mitral valve, the lungs become blown up and congested with blood (Figure 38). The patient then experiences difficulty in breathing because of the stiff lungs. Since his lungs are stuffed with blood under increased pressure, he may also cough up blood.

Left atrium

Narrowed mitral valve

Congested lung

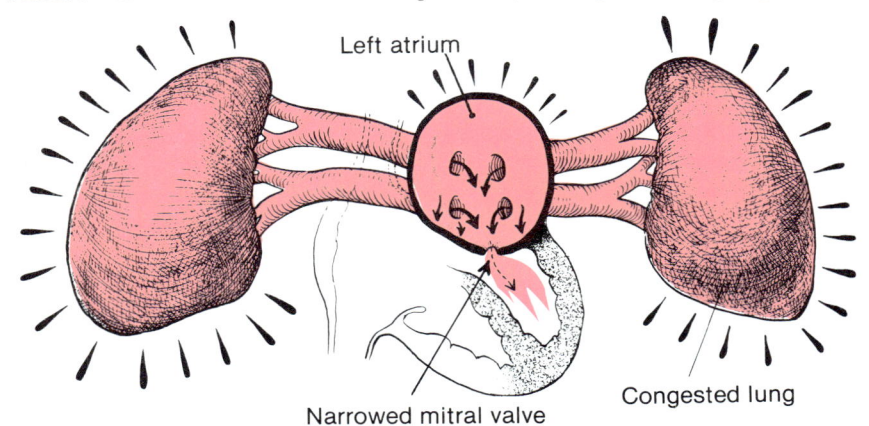

Figure 38 Diagram of the heart and lungs showing the effect of mitral stenosis upon the circulation. The narrowed mitral valve obstructs the free flow of blood from the lungs, which consequently become congested or engorged with blood.

Surgery and Your Heart

This condition is not difficult to treat. It is generally possible for the surgeon to separate the fused edges of the leaflets, so that the blood can again flow freely into the left ventricle (Figure 39). The congestion of the lungs disappears and the patient is no longer breathless.

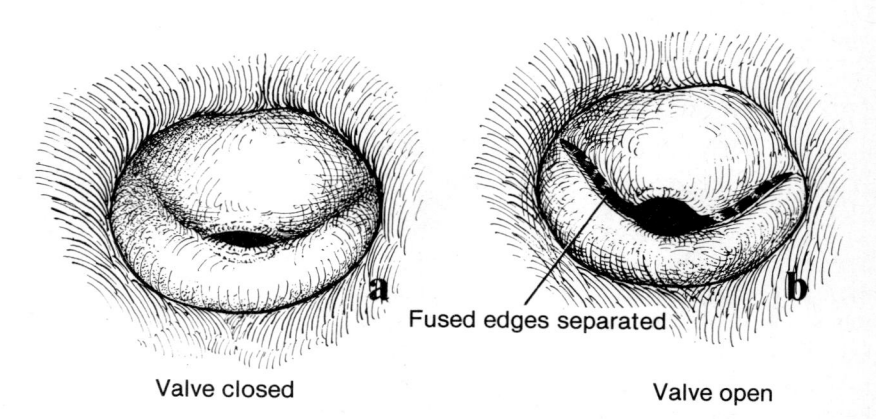

Valve closed   Fused edges separated   Valve open

Figure 39   This drawing of a stenotic mitral valve (a) shows the effects of valvotomy or opening at surgery (b), which allows blood to flow freely through the valve. This relieves the pressure on the lungs.

Aortic Stenosis   Aortic stenosis, caused either by rheumatic fever or the chalky deposits of calcific aortic stenosis, is more dangerous than mitral stenosis. This is because the important high-pressure left ventricle is obstructed by the narrowed valve and pressure builds up in this chamber (Figure 40). The left ventricle has to work much harder to force enough blood into the arteries of the body and, as a result, this overworked pumping chamber thickens progressively and then fails. The patient becomes acutely ill with heart failure.

It is important to recognise this condition before the heart failure becomes irreversible. Also it is usually not possible to split the valve open as with the mitral valve. The narrowed or stenosed aortic valve usually has to be removed, and replaced with a valve made either of biological tissues or plastic and metal (Figure 41). A discussion of the different types of valves used in valve replacement operations follows this chapter.

Diseases of the Heart

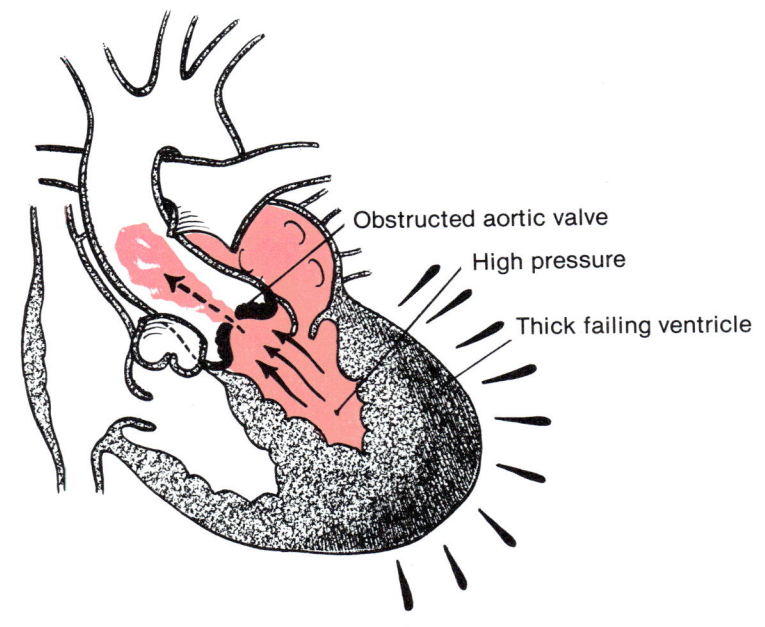

Figure 40 The serious consequences of unrelieved aortic stenosis. The high-pressure left ventricle becomes thick and eventually fails.

Regurgitation of the Mitral or Aortic Valves
When the valves are regurgitant or leaking (Figures 34 and 36), the heart has to work harder by pumping more blood. This compensates for the blood that leaks back through the valve. Thus a regurgitant aortic valve can make the heart enlarge and then fail, and a regurgitant mitral valve has a similar effect, producing congestion in the lungs and heart failure.

The correction of these leaking valves usually involves a valve replacement, although it is sometimes possible to repair them.

Multiple Valve Disease
When more than one valve is diseased, they can be treated at the same time. The treatment of each individual valve will depend upon whether it is stenotic or regurgitant. It may be repaired or replaced depending on the findings at operation.

Surgery and Your Heart

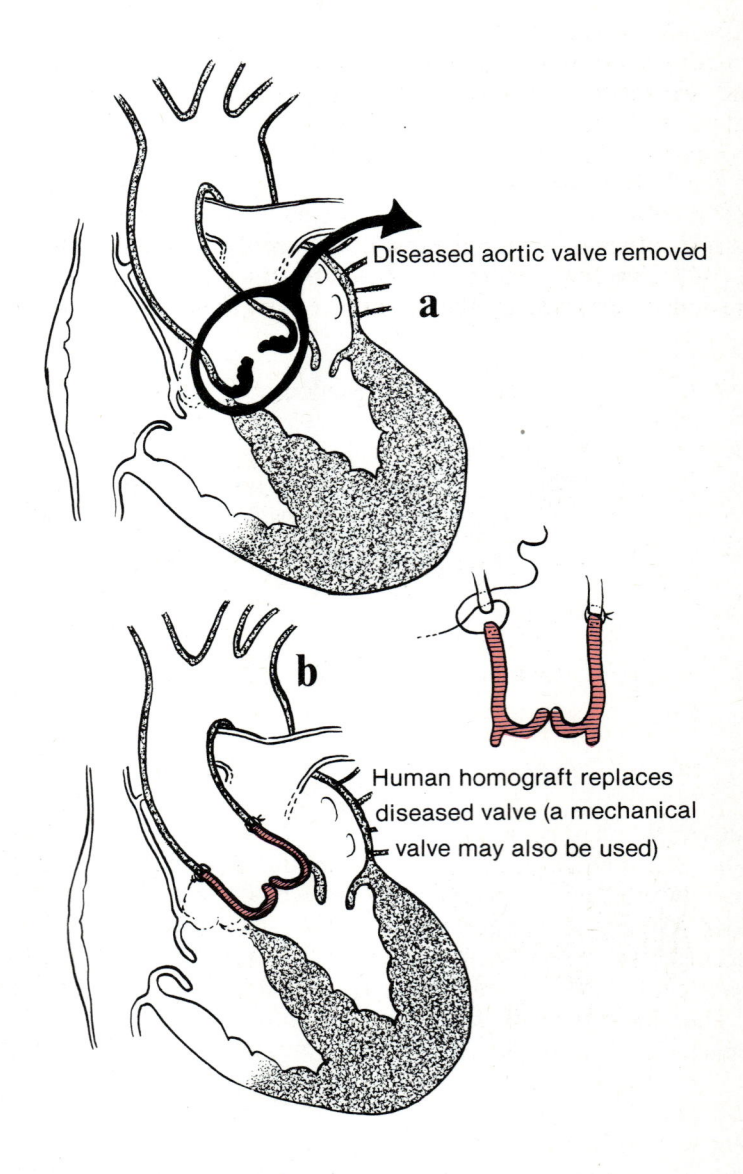

Figure 41   Aortic valve replacement. The diseased aortic valve is removed (a) and a biological or mechanical valve is sewn into its place (b). In this figure the replacement valve is a human homograft.

Diseases of the Heart

Valve Replacement
Valves used to replace the heart's diseased valves come in different sizes and are made of a variety of materials. There are two main types of valves; those made of biological tissues (human or animal tissues), and those made of plastic and metal, called mechanical valves.

The best known tissue valve is the homograft valve. This is a human aortic valve that has been removed from a body shortly after death and then sterilized and stored for use (Figure 42a). It is usually used as an aortic valve replacement, and is sewn in place in the same position previously occupied by the diseased valve (Figure 41). The valve works

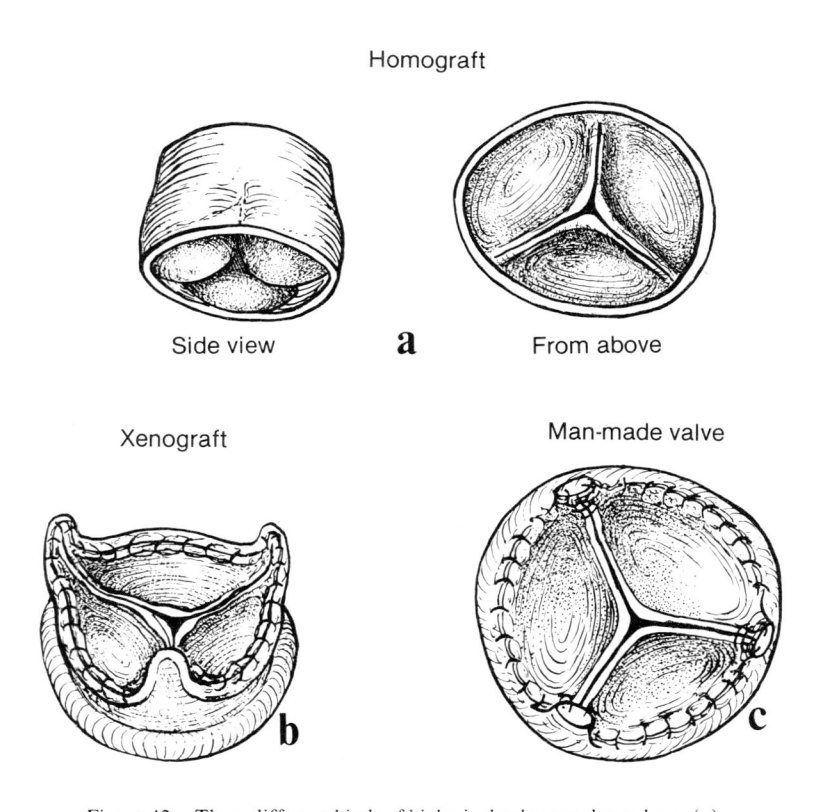

Figure 42 Three different kinds of biological valve are shown here: (a) a homograft – a valve from a human heart, (b) a xenograft – a valve from an animal's heart, and (c) a man-made valve, fashioned out of human or animal tissues (usually pericardium, a tissue which surrounds the heart).

Surgery and Your Heart

well and the patient does not need to take blood-thinning medicines (called anticoagulants), since no blood clots are thrown off from the homograft. The results are very satisfactory from the patient's point of view.

Another type of tissue valve is made from an animal (usually pig) aortic valve sewn onto a flexible frame (Figure 42b). This is called a xenograft, and can be used in almost any valve site. Results with this valve seem to be as good as with the homograft, although they have not been used for as many years.

Figure 42b shows a valve that has been hand made from animal tissue, and sewn onto a frame. The tissue is taken from the membrane surrounding the heart (pericardium) shortly after death, and sterilized and fixed similarly to the xenograft. Again, the results are good for the patient.

Mechanical valves are made of metal, cloth and plastic, and usually are constructed with a design quite different from that of the original valve. This changes the pattern of blood flowing through them, causing turbulence and a tendency for the blood to clot. The mechanical valve in Figure 43 illustrates a common design for an aortic valve, with a moveable ball in a cage. In mechanical mitral valves, the ball is often replaced with a flat disc. The blood flow has to split to flow around the ball or disc, and in this way it differs from the normal flow pattern as seen through a homograft or xenograft valve.

The advantage of mechanical valves is that they are easy to sew in place and are long-lasting. The disadvantage is that they damage the blood and are liable to cause blood clots – because of this, the patient must take blood-thinning medicines (anticoagulants) for the rest of his life. The appropriate dosage of anticoagulants is checked with a blood test every two weeks. Mechanical valves may also be noisy but the patient quickly gets used to them.

The surgeon must weigh the advantages and disadvantages of the various valves, taking into consideration the patient's age, life style and other relevant factors. For example, an active stomach or duodenal ulcer makes the use of anticoagulants hazardous and a biological valve is indicated.

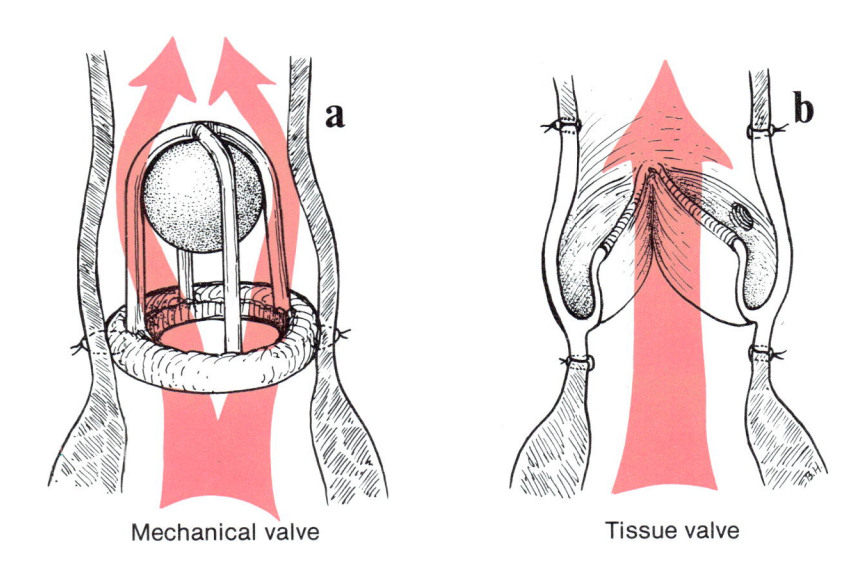

Figure 43 Diagram to show the different flow pattern between (a) a mechanical valve, and (b) a tissue valve (in this case a homograft). The flow pattern is normal in the tissue valve, i.e. centrally flowing, but it is abnormal in the mechanical valve.

Chapter 3
Special Investigations

The examination of the patient with heart disease includes taking his history, examining the pulse, measuring the blood pressure and listening to the heart with a stethoscope. It is usual to have a chest X-ray, which shows the outline of the heart, and to do an electrocardiogram, which shows details of the electrical wave that passes through the heart muscle. Additional special investigations may be necessary to make the diagnosis certain, depending on the disease.

The X-ray

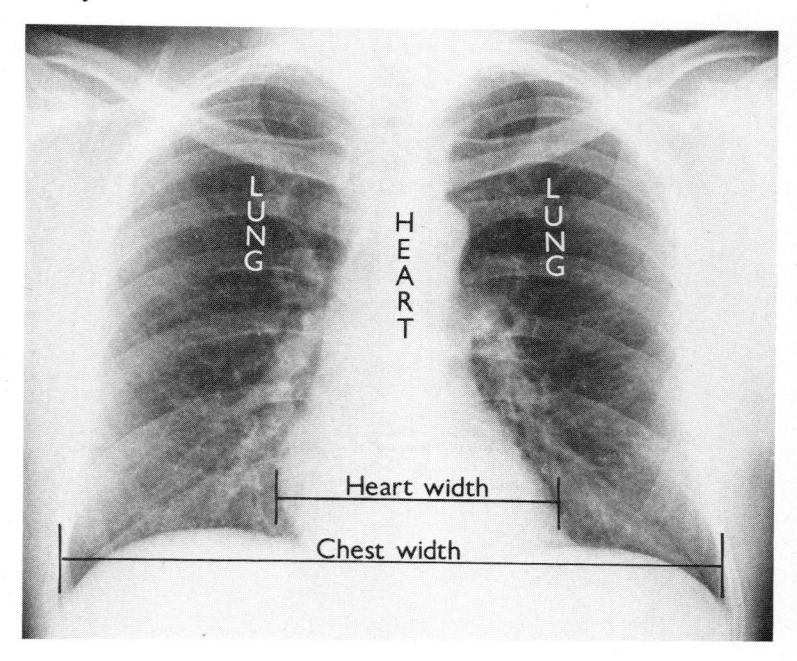

Figure 44 An X-ray of the chest, showing the heart and lungs. The heart shadow is normally less than one half the total width of the chest cavity, as shown here by the markers.

Special Investigations

The chest X-ray gives the doctor valuable information about the patient's heart. First it shows the size of the heart (Figure 44). This is normally less than half the width of the chest cavity. It can also show enlargement of a chamber or chambers of the heart, whether the lungs are congested (as in some forms of valve disease), or whether not enough blood is getting to the lungs (e.g. pulmonary stenosis).

The Electrocardiogram

The electrocardiogram is a tracing of the electrical current which passes through the heart and stimulates the chambers to contract (Figure 45). The doctor can measure the time it takes for certain activities in the heart to occur, and can see how strong the electrical impulses are. It is particularly useful in diagnosing various irregularities in the heart's rhythm, and can indicate which side of the heart is overworking. Heart muscle damage also shows up.

Sometimes a patient may be asked to exercise as an electrical tracing is made. This 'exercise electrocardiogram' shows the rhythm of the heart as it speeds up during the exercise, and shows whether enough blood is reaching the heart muscle. This can serve as a warning of the possible danger of a future heart attack.

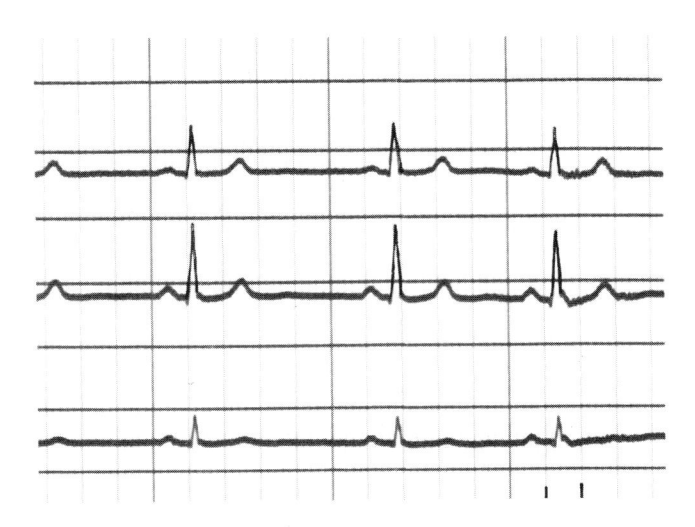

Figure 45 An electrocardiogram, showing the electrical activity which precedes the heart beat.

The Echocardiogram

The echocardiogram is one of the more recent special investigations. The test is carried out quite simply and painlessly by putting a sophisticated little instrument on the patient's chest. This instrument transmits sound waves through the chest wall and the various layers of the heart. A recording is made of the various tissues in the heart as the sound waves bounce off the solid tissues and are reflected back to the instrument. The recording appears on a television-like screen, enabling the doctor to see the various walls and valves of the heart as the heart contracts.

This entirely safe test gives a great deal of information about the size of the heart's chambers and about the action of the individual heart valves. Figure 46 is a tracing taken from the television screen and shows the various layers of the heart through which the sound waves have passed. Nowadays a moving picture can be recorded to show the heart in action.

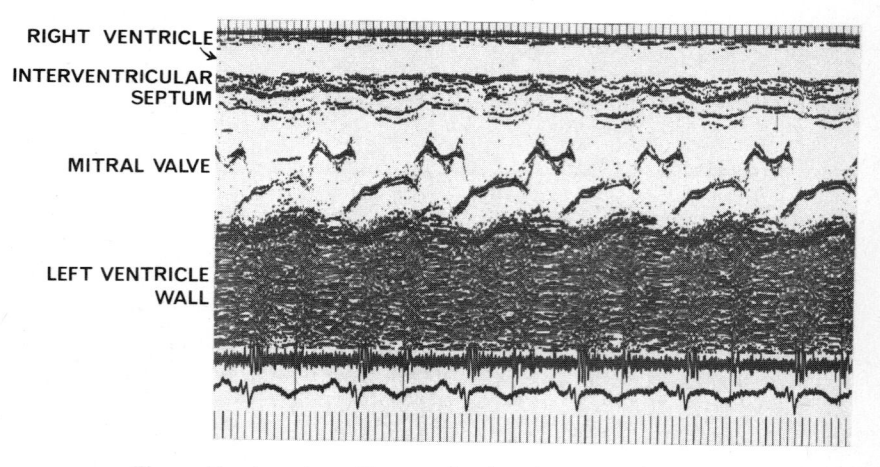

Figure 46 An echocardiogram showing the layers of tissue which reflect the sound waves. The black markings represent solid tissue, the white represents the spaces in the chambers of the heart.

Special Investigations

Cardiac Catheterization and Angiocardiography

These investigations are the most important in the pre-operative diagnosis of heart disease and are often done together. They are not always necessary, but are essential before coronary artery surgery and in most cases of congenital heart disease. The investigation calls for skills and complex apparatus, so that it is always carried out in a hospital or clinic. The procedure is safe and causes the patient little discomfort.

The investigation involves passing a thin hollow tube, called a catheter, through a vein or artery in the arm, into the heart under X-ray and television control (Figure 47). Pressures and blood samples are taken from the various heart chambers for analysis. This is especially important for diagnosing congenital heart disease, since it can tell how much mixed blue and red blood is in a particular chamber, and also measures the pressure in each chamber to see if it is obstructed.

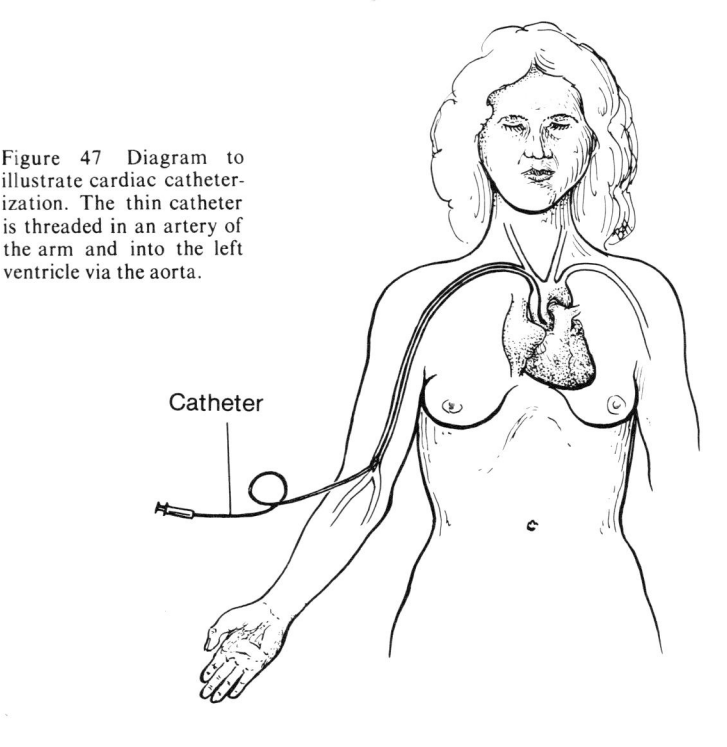

Figure 47 Diagram to illustrate cardiac catheterization. The thin catheter is threaded in an artery of the arm and into the left ventricle via the aorta.

Catheter

Surgery and Your Heart

Angiocardiography is usually done at the same time, and involves the injection of a chemical which shows up on the X-ray and outlines the inside of the heart and great arteries (Figure 48). A movie camera photographs the dye as it passes through the heart chambers. The film can be studied later in a moving projector. Among the many abnormalities that the film can show are:

1) An abnormal pattern of the circulation through the heart, as in congenital heart diseases like transposition of the great vessels,
2) Blood being obstructed by a narrowing or stenosis, as in certain types of valve disease,
3) Blood filling an abnormal space, such as an aneurysm.

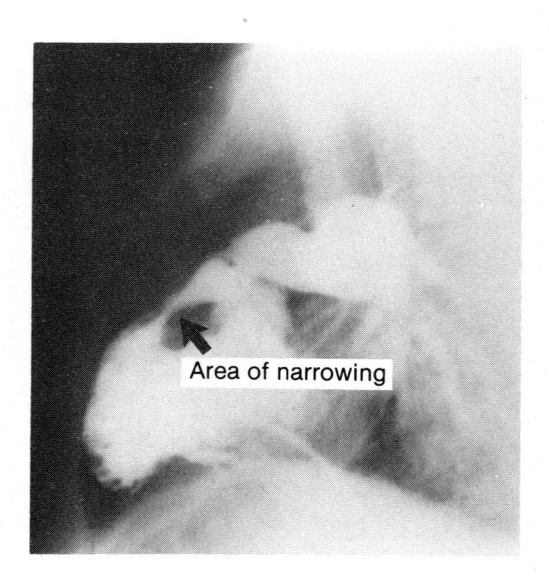

Figure 48   An angiocardiogram showing, in this case, a narrowed area in the pulmonary artery (arrow). This is a side view of the heart.

Special Investigations

Coronary angiography is the same method applied to the study of the coronary arteries. Small amounts of the dye are injected through a catheter inserted directly into the coronary arteries. On the film, the surgeon can see the obstructions or narrowings that cause coronary artery disease or result from a heart attack (Figure 49).

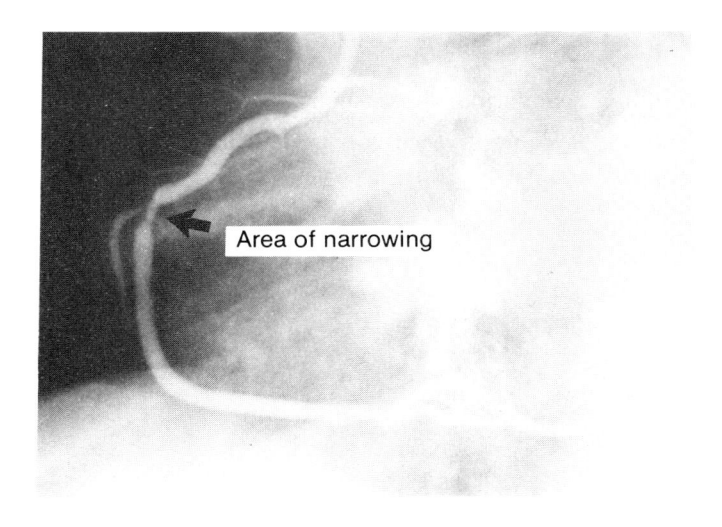

Figure 49   A coronary arteriogram showing a narrowed right coronary artery.

Chapter 4
The Open Heart Operation and Recovery

The Open Heart Operation

Because most heart operations involve opening the heart or major blood vessels, the blood which enters must be redirected to a 'heart-lung machine' while the surgery is carried out. Once the blood is out of the surgical field, the surgeon can see the structures he has to repair.

The patient is connected to the heart-lung machine before opening the heart. This machine takes over the function of the heart and lungs throughout the operation (Figure 50). The tubes which connect the patient to the heart-lung machine are placed in the great veins so that all the blue blood usually entering the heart will flow into the machine instead. Another tube is placed in the aorta so that the oxygenated blood from the machine can be returned to the body, having bypassed the heart. Oxygen is supplied by an artificial lung or oxygenator.

Once the patient is connected to the machine, no blood enters the heart. With the dry heart conditions provided, the surgeon can safely open the heart and make the necessary repairs without danger of losing blood. After the repair, great care is taken to get rid of all air from the various chambers of the heart, and it is gradually allowed to resume its pumping activity. When the heart is again pumping blood, the heart-lung machine is stopped and its connecting tubes are withdrawn. The surgeon can then close the chest incision.

After the Operation

Once the wound is closed, it may be an hour or more before the patient is safe to move. He is then taken to the intensive care ward and kept asleep, and is connected to various machines and measuring instruments. An artificial breathing machine helps the patient breathe while he is unconscious, and electronic measuring instruments record on a screen the electrical activity of the heart and the patient's blood pressure. Also, there are tubes for giving nourishment and fluids, and others for measuring the

The Open Heart Operation and Recovery

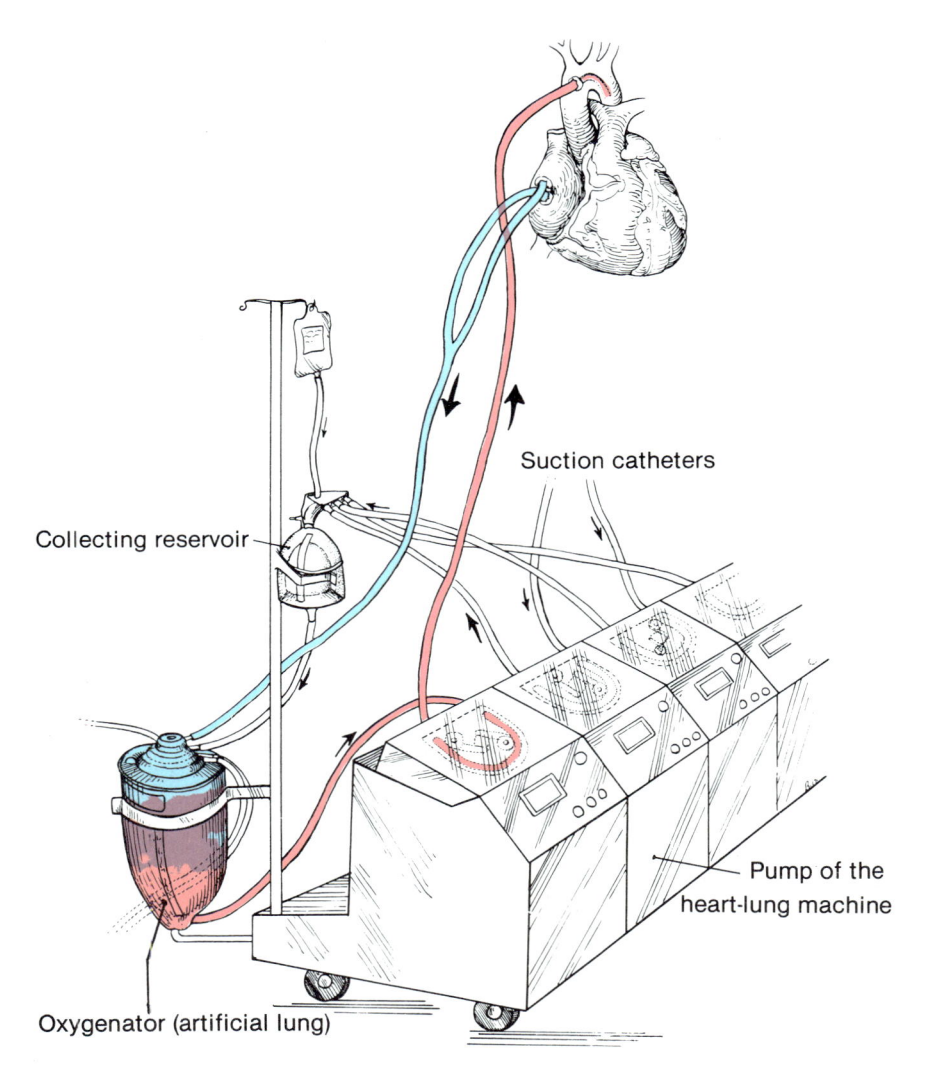

Figure 50 Diagram of the heart-lung machine connected to the heart. Blue blood flows from the veins entering the heart to the oxygenator or artificial lung, where it receives oxygen. From there it goes to the main pump, which pumps it back to the body through a tube (red) that is connected to the aorta. In this way the blood bypasses the heart, so that the surgeon can work in a dry field. The other tubes in the diagram are sucking blood from the area of the operation and returning it to the circulation.

loss of fluids and urine. Samples of blood are taken at regular intervals for analysis.

The patient is kept in the intensive care ward for 24–48 hours, whilst all the measurements are carefully observed and recorded. He is conscious but kept under sedation until the breathing machine, the recorders and various tubes are removed. He then returns to his room.

Post-operative Programme

The First Ten Days
The ten-day period after open heart surgery is usually spent in the clinic or hospital. The first 24–48 hours are spent in the intensive care ward, as described above. By the third day, the patient is usually getting out of bed and may walk around his room.

At this stage there is often a feeling of well-being and relief at being over the operation. Also there is the prospect of being fit again. This mood sometimes amounts to a feeling of euphoria.

It is equally common for this to be followed by a period of reaction or depression, which may set in 3–5 days after the operation. The patient may feel quite depressed, and complains of feeling tired, weak and lacking in appetite. This cycle of events is usual and it is only necessary to explain to the patient that this is everyone's experience, that nothing has gone wrong, and that he should leave matters to nature to resolve. This applies particularly to the appetite, and nothing is to be gained by anxious relatives pleading with the patient to eat.

Normally, by 7–10 days, the patient feels quite well and has by then been walked down the corridors and up a few stairs in preparation for leaving the clinic. Aches and pains felt in the region of the wound or the shoulders and base of the neck, as well as a slight temperature, are a result of the healing reaction around the heart. Aspirin compounds and reassurance are the prescribed treatment here.

Continuity of care is important for a patient, and it is ideal if the doctor or practitioner who will attend the patient later, at home or in the hotel, visits the patient while still in the hospital or clinic. He can familiarise himself with the patient's post-operative course, and the patient, in turn, will know that he has someone to turn to outside the hospital or clinic.

At the time the patient leaves the hospital, he will be given any necessary medicines and simple instructions about his early convalescence. He is given an appointment to visit his surgeon and

The Open Heart Operation and Recovery

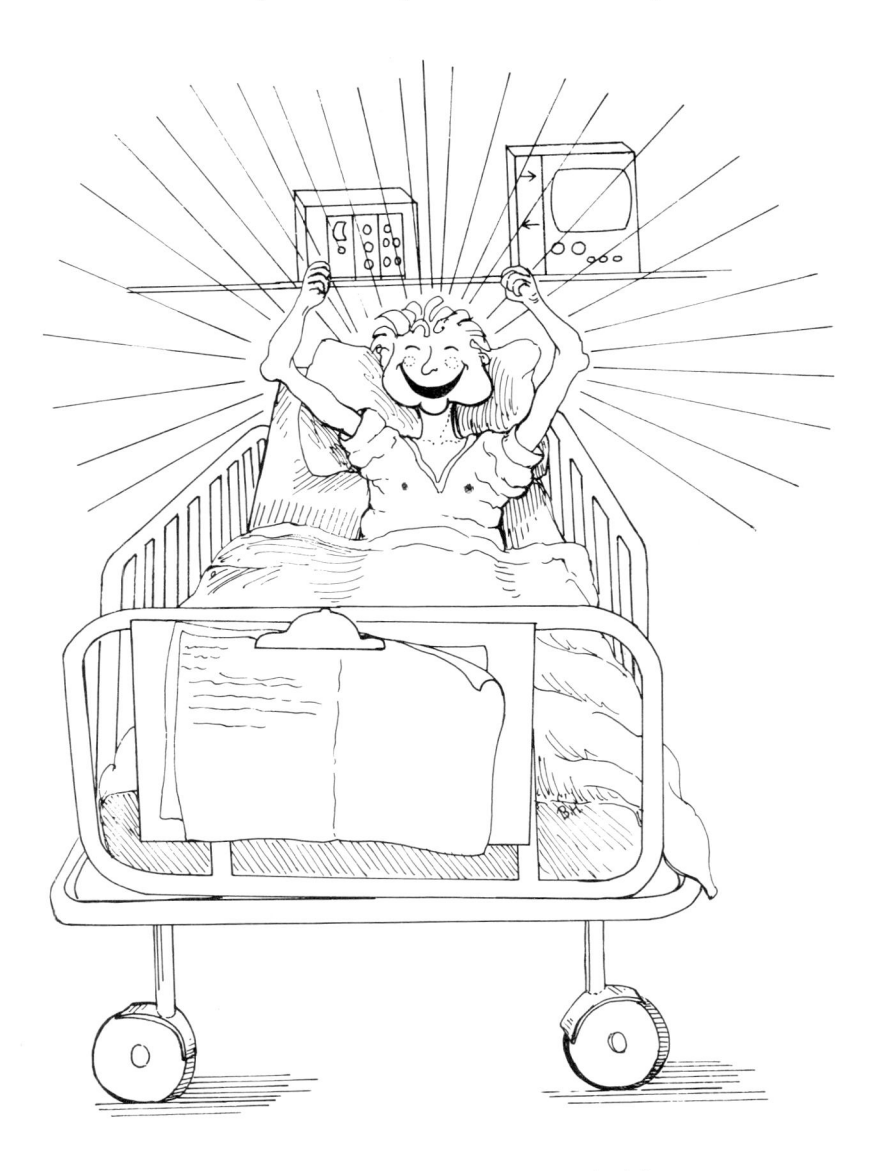

Figure 51 Recovery days 1 and 2: euphoria!

Surgery and Your Heart

cardiologist about 7–10 days after leaving the hospital, and appointments are also made for his blood check, electrocardiogram and chest X-ray.

If problems arise once the patient has left the hospital, he can contact the general practitioner who is already familiar with his case and he, in turn, will contact the patient's cardiologist or surgeon if this is necessary.

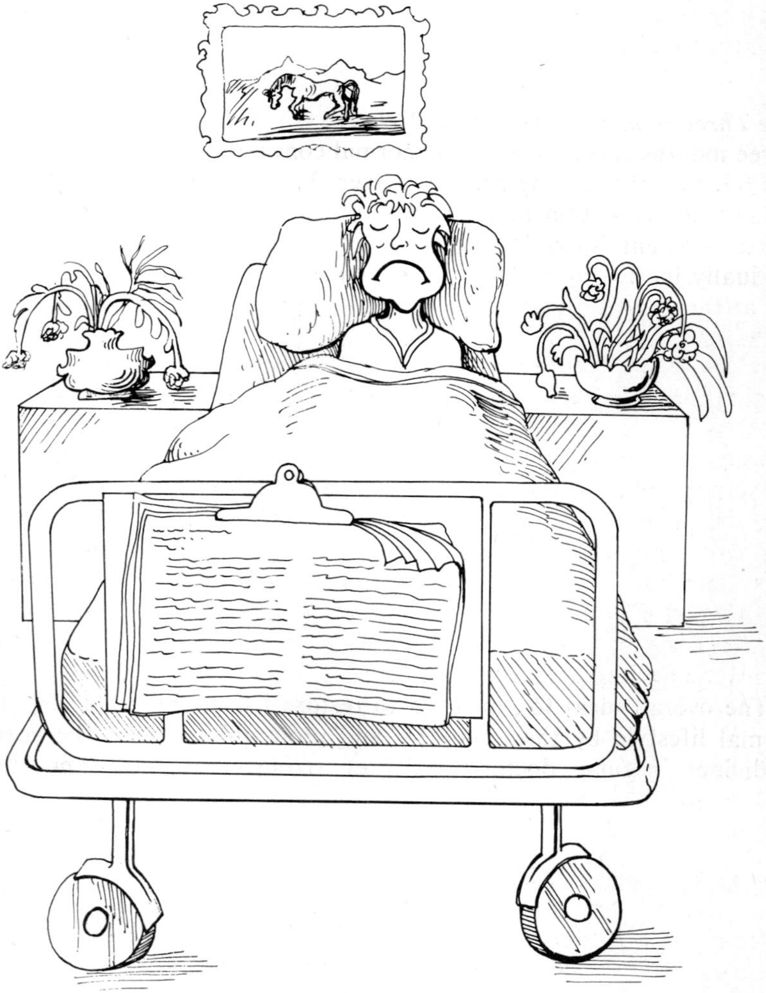

Figure 52 Recovery days 3 to 5: depression.

The Open Heart Operation and Recovery

When the patient reattends his cardiologist and surgeon, his blood, chest X-ray and electrocardiogram will be studied, as well as the healing of his wound and the condition of the heart. Any change in medication will be made at that time, and further instructions will be given to cover the three-month period after the surgery. At this time reports will be sent to the patient's doctor describing the operation in detail, together with the post-operative programme, medication and relevant advice about the patient's future.

The Three-month Convalescent Period

Three months is regarded as the normal convalescent period, after which it is felt that the healing process is over. The patient is often able to stop all or most medication, and return to a normal active life.

The patient should spend the three-month convalescent period gradually increasing his activities, with a view to living a normal active life at the end of that time. Any activity or exertion including walking, sunbathing and swimming should be encouraged, as long as the patient feels well and enjoys the activity. No attempt should be made to adhere to a rigid pattern, but again nature should be the guide to activity and diet.

Many patients and their relatives are over-concerned with their diet at this stage, and with how to modify it to prevent further problems. During the important convalescent period when the body is repairing itself, no attempt should be made to adhere to a strict diet. Instead, the patient should eat and drink in moderation exactly what he enjoys, until the body's physical state is again normal. After the three months the patient's own doctor may advise or impose a way of life designed to prevent a recurrence of the disease process, but this should not be rigidly adopted before the healing process is complete.

The overall ideal to aim at is to restore the patient to a completely normal lifestyle by three months, and preferably without the need for medicines, regular doctor's visits or stringent physical and dietary restrictions.

Eating, Drinking and Smoking

Most patients are aware of the importance of diet as a cause of, say, coronary artery disease, and there is good evidence for this. For instance, the disease is uncommon in the rice-eating people of the East, and very common in the West, where meat and fats predominate in the diet. A sensible attitude therefore is to reduce the intake of meat and fats, and increase the vegetable content of our diets. This additional bulk in the food has added advantages in maintaining our health and well-being, and has even been suggested as a factor in protecting us from bowel cancer. The patient should try to shift the emphasis away from a high intake of meat, eggs and fatty foods. It is not necessary to remove these foods completely from the diet.

It should be realised that the disease process is a slowly developing one, probably over a number of years, and a sudden change of dietary habits post-operatively will not bring about a dramatic improvement in the health of our blood vessels. The diet should provide a sensible change in intake and character, designed to reduce the fat intake and to avoid becoming overweight. The programme should be looked upon as a long-term change of habits spread over 5–10 years, and include regular exercise as a part of the plan. A salt-free diet is rarely necessary, but added salt should be avoided.

Smoking and alcohol are often implicated in coronary artery disease. Smoking certainly makes the pain of coronary artery disease worse, probably by causing spasm of the small arteries, and there is additional evidence to suggest that it may be a factor in causing the disease. On the other hand, alcohol, in moderation, has a gentle dilating effect on the arteries, and may in fact be beneficial.

Regular exercise should be encouraged, especially walking and swimming, but in the case of young children with congenital heart disease, competitive sports should usually be discouraged for one year.

Similarly, pregnancy should be avoided for one year after surgery and the patient's doctor should advise on the use of contraceptive pills.

The teeth are a source of danger to all patients who have had heart surgery, and infections of the teeth may enter the bloodstream at the time of dental extractions or any other dental treatment. It is vitally important to notify the dentist about the recent heart surgery, and to ensure that appropriate antibiotics are taken to protect against bloodstream infections which may settle on the operation area.

The patient's aftercare is in the hands of his own doctor, but it is an advantage for the cardiologist and surgeon to have annual reports on his progress for their records. With congenital and valve disease there should be a regular review of the patient's condition at intervals of 1–2 years.

The Open Heart Operation and Recovery

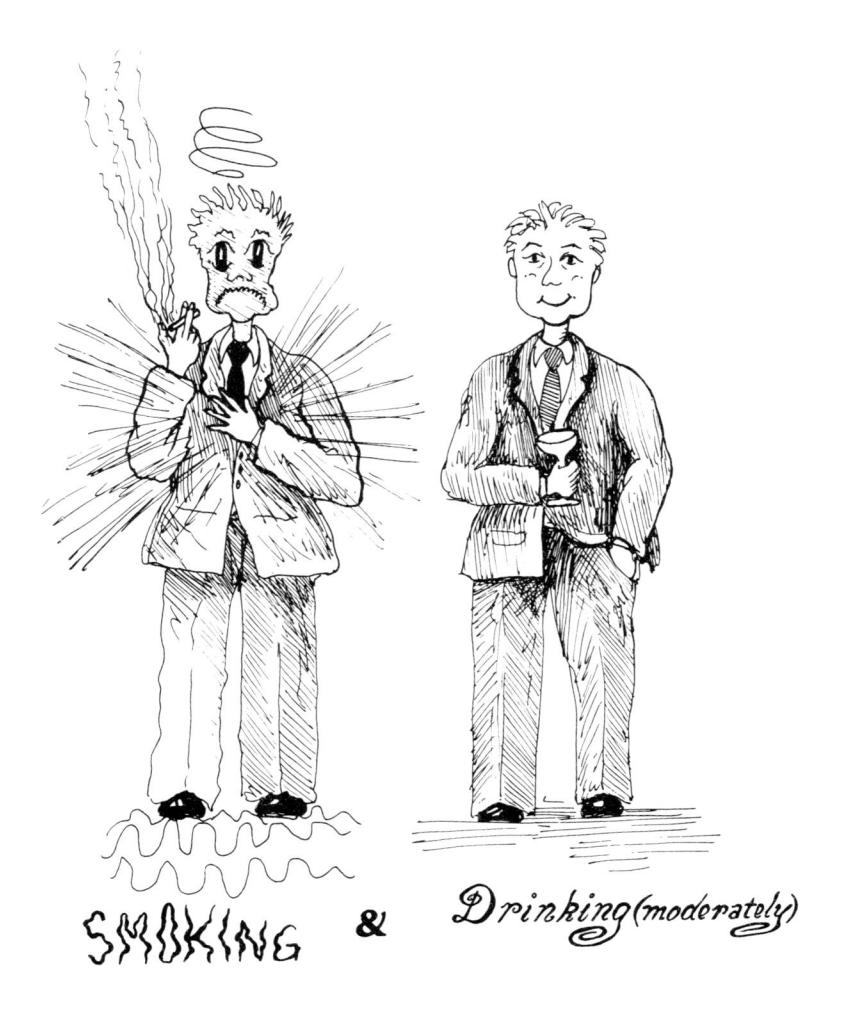

Figure 53 Smoking and drinking – smoking makes the pain of coronary artery disease worse, whereas alcohol in moderation is permissible.

Other books by Mr Donald Ross

A Surgeon's Guide to Cardiac Diagnosis
Part I: The Diagnostic Approach, 1962
Part II: The Clinical Picture, 1967
Springer-Verlag

Medical and Surgical Cardiology
Jointly with William Cleland, John Goodwin and Lawson McDonald
Blackwell Scientific Publications, 1969

Biological Tissue in Heart Valve Replacement
Edited by M. I. Ionescu, D. N. Ross and G. H. Wooler
Butterworth, 1972

Other books illustrated by Ms Barbara Hyams

Techniques in Cardiac Surgery
Denton A. Cooley and John C. Norman
T. C. Hengst, co-illustrator
Texas Medical Press, 1975

Techniques in Vascular Surgery
Denton A. Cooley and Don C. Wukasch
T. C. Hengst and R. G. Jones, co-illustrators
W. B. Saunders, 1979